Dear Reader,

I think most of us can agree that we want our lives to be filled with energy and good health as we get older. And with a wide body of evidence behind it, the Mediterranean diet **offers a lot** when it comes to reducing the risk of developing chronic diseases as we age. Taking it one step further, the MIND diet blends all the research we know about the Mediterranean diet and pulls in all of the health benefits of the DASH diet (Dietary Approaches to Stop Hypertension). The goal: Reduce the risk of developing Alzheimer's and other age-related cognitive decline.

The highlight of the MIND diet is enjoying foods that are vibrant on the plate, rich in antioxidants and anti-inflammatory compounds, and loaded with fiber. All things that are both attractive to eat and nourishing to **your mind and body**. It is important to note that a traditional Mediterranean diet may not seem appealing to everyone or may not be culturally representative. This is why you will see this often referred to as a Mediterranean-style diet.

The focus of the MIND diet is on fruits, vegetables, beans, legumes, fish and other sources of omega-3 fatty acids, whole grains, nuts, and lean meats. Swapping ingredients that are more culturally representative for your heritage is a great way to honor your culture while reaping the benefits of the MIND diet. For example, sardines and anchovies are popular in traditional Mediterranean diets, but less so in the US, so we frequently recommend salmon instead. The goals with nutrients won't change and a **variety of foods** can be used to meet the MIND diet needs for fruits, vegetables, whole grains, beans, lentils, and nuts, along with sources of omega-3s. Hence, a Mediterranean-style diet, like the MIND diet, can work for anyone! The recipes found in this cookbook are sure to be a hit in any home with people who are looking to keep their minds sharp without feeling deprived of flavor.

Melinda Boyd, DCN, RD, FAND

Welcome to the Everything® Series!

These handy, accessible books give you all you need to tackle a difficult project, gain a new hobby, comprehend a fascinating topic, prepare for an exam, or even brush up on something you learned back in school but have since forgotten.

You can choose to read an Everything® book from cover to cover or just pick out the information you want from our four useful boxes: Questions, Facts, Alerts, and Essentials. We give you everything you need to know on the subject, but throw in a lot of fun stuff along the way too.

question

Answers to common questions.

fact

Important snippets of information.

alert

Urgent warnings.

essential

Quick handy tips.

We now have more than 600 Everything® books in print, spanning such wide-ranging categories as cooking, health, parenting, personal finance, wedding planning, word puzzles, and so much more. When you're done reading them all, you can finally say you know Everything®!

PUBLISHER Karen Cooper

MANAGING EDITOR Lisa Laing

ASSOCIATE COPY DIRECTOR Casey Ebert

PRODUCTION EDITOR Jo-Anne Duhamel

SENIOR ACQUISITIONS EDITOR Julia Belkas

SENIOR DEVELOPMENT EDITOR Brett Palana-Shanahan

EVERYTHING® SERIES COVER DESIGNER Erin Alexander

THE EVERYTHING® *Easy* MIND Diet Cookbook

175 Delicious Recipes to Combat Dementia, Improve Cognitive Function, and Support Overall Health

Christy Ellingsworth
With Melinda Boyd, DCN, RD, FAND

ADAMS MEDIA
NEW YORK AMSTERDAM/ANTWERP LONDON TORONTO
SYDNEY/MELBOURNE NEW DELHI

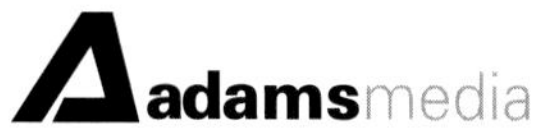

Adams Media
An Imprint of Simon & Schuster, LLC
100 Technology Center Drive
Stoughton, MA 02072

An Everything® Series Book.

Everything® and everything.com® are registered trademarks of Simon & Schuster, LLC.

First Adams Media trade paperback edition
May 2026

ADAMS MEDIA and colophon are registered trademarks of Simon & Schuster, LLC.

Interior layout by Maya Caspi
Photographs by Emily Weeks

Manufactured in the United States of America

1 2026

Library of Congress Control Number: 2025949311

ISBN 978-1-5072-2640-7
ISBN 978-1-5072-2641-4 (ebook)

Contains material adapted from the following titles published by Adams Media, an Imprint of Simon & Schuster, LLC: *The Everything® Guide to the MIND Diet* by Christy Ellingsworth and Murdoc Khaleghi, MD, copyright © 2016, ISBN 978-1-4405-9799-2, and *The Everything® DASH Diet Cookbook* by Christy Ellingsworth and Murdoc Khaleghi, MD, copyright © 2012, ISBN 978-1-4405-4353-1.

Contents

Introduction

If you are reading this cookbook, it's likely that you or a loved one has experienced some form of cognitive decline or has been diagnosed with Alzheimer's disease. Or perhaps you've heard about the benefits of the MIND diet in improving your brain health and want to set yourself on the best possible path for your future well-being. Whatever the reason, you've come to the right place. Preventing Alzheimer's disease, dementia, and other forms of cognitive decline may be as simple as making better food choices. Fortunately, with the recipes and information found throughout *The Everything® Easy MIND Diet Cookbook*, you can help fight cognitive decline and improve your overall health.

The MIND diet—short for Mediterranean-DASH Intervention for Neurodegenerative Delay—attempts to reverse mental decline. The MIND diet focuses on adopting foods that can protect the brain and steers you away from foods that could do damage to your body and brain health.

The simplicity of the MIND diet is that it allows you to eat many types of foods while only discouraging a few types. Rather than having to be overly restrictive, you merely have to direct yourself toward more healthful choices—and with the recipes throughout this book, those choices will be easy to make! The 175 recipes in this book will help you enjoy delicious foods that not only fulfill your cravings but keep you feeling healthy and well.

From memory-boosting breakfasts and enticing dinners to desserts of all kinds, the recipes in this book are diverse, delicious, and easy to prepare—and best of all, they require only simple, everyday ingredients, so you don't have to spend your valuable time running out to the store. With step-by-step instructions and handy tips and suggestions, eating on the MIND diet has never been easier!

Inside, you'll find new, healthier versions of your favorite foods that you'll want to make again and again, such as:

- Gingerbread Pancakes
- Glazed Balsamic Chicken Wings
- Salmon with Mango and Chickpea Salad
- Seared Sirloin Steaks with Garlicky Greens
- Homemade Black Bean Burgers
- Peanut Butter Chocolate Chip Blondies
- Maple Mocha Frappé
- And so much more!

In addition, you'll also find a chapter that delves into the acceptable foods and foods to avoid (or limit your consumption of) on this diet and shows you the role food plays in memory and health. You'll learn about the vitamins, nutrients, and other essential elements your body and brain need to function at their peak performance. At the end of the book, you'll also find helpful meal plans to make eating on the MIND diet even easier.

Whether you are new to the MIND diet or just looking for new brain-healthy ideas, you'll find plenty of delicious recipes in this book along with valuable information to help you take charge of your health journey. Eating on the MIND diet doesn't mean missing out on your favorite foods or fun events—it simply means making small, meaningful dietary changes that will support your brain health, and overall health, now and into the future.

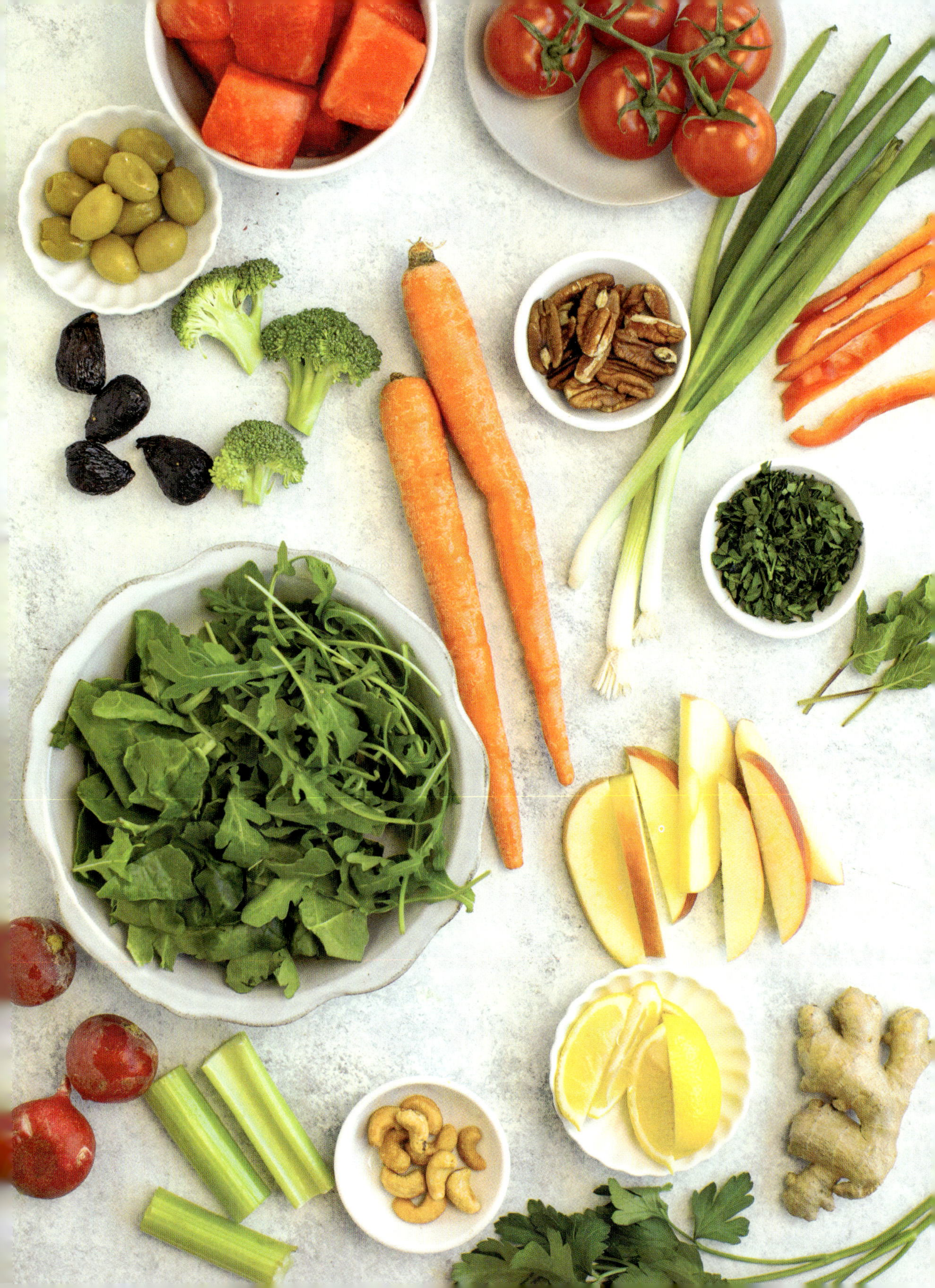

CHAPTER 1

What Is the MIND Diet?

The MIND diet emphasizes the consumption of plant-based foods and healthy fats while limiting the consumption of animal products and foods that are high in saturated fat. In addition to the healthy fats, there is also an emphasis on green leafy vegetables and berries. This way of eating has been proven to reduce the risk of Alzheimer's disease and fight the effects of aging on the brain. In this chapter you'll learn how and why the MIND diet was developed as well as the foods that are included and excluded on the diet. You'll also discover how Alzheimer's disease and dementia affect your brain and how the foods on the MIND diet specifically help keep your brain working at its best for years to come.

The History of the MIND Diet

In February 2015, a study was published in the medical journal *Alzheimer's & Dementia* that intrigued and surprised readers. According to the researchers, older adults who followed a specific diet, called the Mediterranean-DASH Intervention for Neurodegenerative Delay diet, or the MIND diet, were able to reduce their risk of developing Alzheimer's disease—and rather significantly. Study participants who followed the MIND diet "moderately well" showed a 35 percent reduction in risk of developing Alzheimer's disease, but those who strictly adhered to it saw even better results. In fact, the study participants who followed the diet to the letter saw reductions in Alzheimer's disease risk of up to 53 percent.

Dr. Martha Clare Morris, a nutritional epidemiologist at Rush University Medical Center, developed the MIND diet. Her study in 2015 was funded by the National Institute on Aging, and followed the food intake of 923 Chicago-area senior citizens over a period of four and a half years. After this time, researchers found that 144 of the study participants developed Alzheimer's disease while the remaining study participants did not. The researchers concluded that the longer and more closely participants followed the diet, the less risk they had of developing Alzheimer's disease and other cognitive impairments.

Your Brain and Alzheimer's Disease

Before we dive deeper into how food plays a role in your memory and the health of your brain in general, let's take a quick look at what Alzheimer's disease and dementia are—and the known risk factors for developing them.

alert

More than 7 million Americans are living with Alzheimer's disease or another form of dementia. Alzheimer's disease is currently the sixth-leading cause of death in the United States. The disease kills more people than prostate cancer and breast cancer combined.

Your brain contains about 100 billion nerve cells, called neurons. Each one of these neurons connects with many others to form communication networks all over the brain and the rest of your body. Some of these neurons are involved in thinking, learning, and remembering past events and new information, while others help you move or see or smell. Your brain is the control center of your body, and in order for it to work properly there must be flawless communication between all of these neural networks.

Researchers have identified some risk factors that increase the likelihood of developing Alzheimer's disease and other neurodegenerative disorders, but there are still a lot of questions that remain unanswered. One thing that researchers do agree on, however, is that somewhere, somehow, neurons become damaged and are unable to do their job. As the damage spreads, more cells become affected and some begin to die off. It's the death of these nerve cells that causes the symptoms that are characteristic of Alzheimer's disease.

Alzheimer's Disease and Dementia

Dementia is not a specific disease; it's a general term that describes a decline in memory, thinking skills, and cognition that is severe enough to interfere with a person's ability to perform normal, everyday activities. Alzheimer's disease, which is the most common form of dementia, accounts for 60–80 percent of cases. While symptoms of dementia and Alzheimer's disease can vary from person to person, some of the most common include:

- Impaired memory
- Reduced communication and language skills
- Inability to focus
- Decrease in reasoning and judgment
- Impaired visual perception

Most forms of dementia are progressive, which means the symptoms start out gradual and then get worse as time goes on.

The greatest known risk factor for developing dementia and Alzheimer's disease is advancing age. One out of nine people aged sixty-five or older have Alzheimer's; one out of three aged eighty-five or older are affected. Another known risk factor for Alzheimer's is genetics. If you have a family member who has been affected by Alzheimer's, you are more likely to become affected as well.

While you can't change your heredity or your family history, you can change your lifestyle, which includes the food you're eating. If you eat in a way that prohibits certain genes from expressing themselves, you may be able to prevent diseases like Alzheimer's or even reduce the severity of symptoms once they develop.

Other Benefits of the MIND Diet

When you focus on a diet that's rich in anti-inflammatory, antioxidant-rich foods and devoid of foods that largely contribute to weight gain and inflammation, you'll begin to notice an improvement in all areas of your health. The MIND diet was developed to improve brain health and reduce the risk of Alzheimer's disease and other neurodegenerative disorders, but following the program results in other health benefits as well. The following sections will highlight the other benefits you may find from going on the MIND diet.

Improving Blood Sugar and Insulin Levels

The types of foods that affect your blood sugar levels the most are refined, rapidly digesting carbohydrates, such as white breads, white crackers, white rice, potatoes, sweets, and desserts. The more processed a sugar is, the faster it moves through your digestive system and into your bloodstream. The faster that sugar moves through your digestive system, the more dramatic the resulting spike in blood sugar is.

The MIND diet eliminates these foods and encourages the consumption of slower -digesting carbohydrates like berries, beans, lentils, green leafy vegetables, and nuts. These foods are not only inherently good for your brain; they also help stabilize your blood sugar and insulin levels. Other ways you can keep your blood sugar and insulin levels steady include eating three balanced meals and small snacks throughout the day, avoiding skipping meals, and avoiding overeating.

Reducing the Risk of Cardiovascular Disease

Research shows that Mediterranean-style diets, the type of diet on which the MIND diet is based, can significantly reduce the risk of heart disease. The focus of the diet isn't necessarily on limiting total fat intake (although you should pay some attention to how many calories you're taking in), but rather paying attention to the types of fats you're eating. Olive oil is rich in monounsaturated fats that help lower cholesterol levels, but it is also high in antioxidants that help protect your heart—and the rest of your body. The omega-3 fatty acids in the fish recommended on the MIND diet also help promote healthy blood clotting, reduce triglyceride levels, and improve the health of your blood vessels. They are also associated with a decreased incidence of sudden heart attacks.

essential

Remember you can use your own traditional cultural foods to match the style of the MIND diet by selecting those foods that closely align with the key food group/nutrients recommended on the diet. If there is a suggested food that doesn't appeal to you or is difficult to find in your area, feel free to substitute it for a similarly healthful food.

Strengthening Your Immune System

Your diet plays an integral part in strengthening your immune system—or weakening it if you're eating the wrong types of foods. Research shows that eating a diet high in fruits, vegetables, and whole grains, and low in saturated fats, is one of the first lines of defense against sickness. Certain nutrients are especially good at boosting your immune system, and each one of these nutrients is found in abundance on the MIND diet.

They are:

- Vitamin C
- Vitamin E
- Vitamin D
- Selenium
- Zinc

Reducing Inflammation

Your diet can play a significant role in the amount of inflammation in your body. What you eat can either fuel inflammation or cool it down. The foods that are discouraged from the MIND diet, like red meat, sweets (sugary foods), and fried foods, are highly inflammatory foods, while the foods that are the foundation of the program are anti-inflammatory. Some of the main components of the diet (dark leafy greens, nuts, and whole grains) are especially good for reducing inflammation in the body because they are all rich in magnesium—a mineral that an estimated 60 percent of Americans have insufficient intake of. Research shows that people with high inflammatory markers tend to have low levels of magnesium. There also seems to be a connection between low magnesium and inflammation-related disorders like heart disease and diabetes.

Balancing Digestive Health

The first step to balancing your digestive system is to remove any foods or drinks that could be inflammatory or irritating. The next step is to allow your body to start repairing itself by giving it all of the nutrients it needs to build new, healthy cells. By following the MIND diet, you've already got these first two steps covered. You'll also want to make sure you're drinking enough water to keep you hydrated and your digestive system healthy. For many people, these three steps alone are enough to get the digestive system back on track. For others, supplementation may be necessary. Supplements that are especially good for the digestive system are probiotics and digestive enzymes.

What to Eat on the MIND Diet and Why

The MIND diet is built around fifteen major food categories—ten of these categories are healthy foods that provide the foundation of the diet, and the other five categories are foods that should be avoided or limited while following the plan. The following sections will explore these categories in more depth. In addition to these staple foods, you can also enjoy low-fat yogurt, other legumes like lentils, and other healthy fats like avocado, coconut, and olives as part of your plan. These foods should not take the place of the daily staples, but they are okay to include with your meals.

When Dr. Morris developed the MIND diet, she had two major goals in mind. The first was to create a diet plan that could improve brain health and cut the risk of developing devastating neurodegenerative disorders like Alzheimer's disease significantly. The second was to ensure that the diet was easy to follow, so that people would actually stick to the program and see the results they were after. The MIND diet doesn't have strict daily recommendations for each group or for specific minerals, like sodium. Instead, the MIND diet gives general recommendations that should be followed every day. Following are the daily recommended servings for the foods you should eat on the MIND diet and suggested amounts for the foods you should limit.

Brain-Protecting Foods

The two main underlying factors that lead to neurodegenerative diseases are inflammation and oxidative stress—which happens when the production of free radicals, which come from a poor diet, excess stress, and toxins (like pollution or cigarette smoke) in the body is greater than your body's ability to neutralize those free radicals through antioxidants. In order to prevent neurodegenerative diseases from developing, you have to eliminate chronic inflammation and combat oxidative stress by altering your eating habits. This is the main principle of the MIND diet.

The ten "brain-healthy foods" of the MIND diet provide different nutrients that help boost cognitive function and improve memory and learning skills. The five "brain-unhealthy foods" contribute to cognitive decline and may even play a role in the development of Alzheimer's disease and other forms of dementia. The recommended serving sizes for the ten healthy foods are (in order of importance):

- Green leafy vegetables—at least six servings per week
- Other vegetables—at least one per day
- Nuts—at least five servings per week
- Blueberries—two or more servings per week
- Whole grains—three or more servings per day
- Beans—at least three servings per week
- Fish—at least two serving per week
- Poultry—at least two servings per week
- Olive oil—consume daily (use as your main cooking oil)
- Red wine—one glass (4–5 ounces) per day

Now, let's look at each of these foods in more depth.

Green Leafy Vegetables

Green leafy vegetables are one of the main focuses of the MIND diet—and for good reason. They are loaded with nutrients that perform a wide range of functions to keep you healthy, but there are some specific vitamins that give the greens their brain-boosting power.

In a study led by Morris, researchers tracked the diets and cognitive abilities of 923 older adults (with an average age of eighty-one) for a period of four and a half years. The researchers witnessed a rapid decrease in the rate of cognitive decline in the study participants who consumed the largest amount of leafy green vegetables, which are rich in vitamin K. The study participants who ate one or two servings of leafy greens per day had cognitive abilities equivalent to a person eleven years younger when compared to participants who consumed no leafy greens. Researchers believe that in addition to folate, lutein, and beta-carotene, vitamin K is largely responsible for this effect.

Other Vegetables

Although leafy greens are one of the vegetable powerhouses of the MIND diet program, other vegetables are included in the diet as well. Brightly colored vegetables, like carrots and squash, and cruciferous vegetables, like broccoli and cauliflower, are also loaded with beta-carotene and antioxidants that protect the brain from damage from free radicals and help ward off inflammation, which can put stress on the brain and reduce both short-term and long-term memory.

Nuts

Walnuts are high in alpha-linolenic acid—a plant-based omega-3 fatty acid that is known to ward off Alzheimer's disease. They are also extremely high in antioxidants, which protect against inflammation and cell damage, and magnesium, which can help the heart cope under the pressure of stressful times. It's not just walnuts that are beneficial for brain health, though. Nuts in general are a rich source of vitamin E, an antioxidant-rich, fat-soluble vitamin that helps protect the brain from damage from free radicals.

Blueberries

Blueberries are the only fruit specifically recommended on the MIND diet. The diet doesn't prohibit the consumption of other fruits, but it also doesn't emphasize increased consumption of all fruits. However, blueberries are purposely included in the diet because of their significant brain-boosting power.

Blueberries get their color from a class of compounds called flavonoids. They're especially rich in a specific flavonoid group called anthocyanins. A study published in the journal *Free Radical Biology & Medicine* in 2004 reported that the flavonoids in blueberries are able to cross the blood-brain barrier and interact with the nerve cells (neurons) in the brain, improving communication between the neural networks and stimulating the regeneration of new brain cells. This process can improve both short-term and long-term memory and help increase the ability to retain new information.

Whole Grains

The ability of whole grains to help ward off Alzheimer's disease comes mainly from their fiber content. Whole grains are rich in fiber, which helps slow the digestion and absorption of food through your digestive tract. When digestion is slowed down, it also slows down the release of glucose in your blood. As a result, you don't experience a rapid surge in blood sugar—or the rapid surge in insulin levels that follows.

If your body consistently experiences dramatic increases in blood sugar and insulin, over time it can lead to insulin resistance—a condition in which the body is unable to use insulin effectively. Research shows that insulin resistance could increase the risk of developing Alzheimer's disease by changing the way your brain uses glucose—or sugar—which is its preferred source of energy. When you become insulin resistant, glucose cannot enter the cells effectively, and as a result, your brain—and other parts of your body—can become starved of energy.

Beans

Beans and other legumes, like green peas, are rich in B-complex vitamins, which protect the brain against shrinkage and help to maintain a healthy nervous system. Like whole grains, beans are also rich in fiber, so they can help slow down digestion and keep blood sugar and insulin levels steady.

Fish

Fatty fish, like salmon, are especially high in omega-3 fatty acids. These fatty acids help protect the brain against beta-amyloid—the protein whose presence is linked to higher incidences of Alzheimer's disease. A study published in *Archives of Neurology* found that people aged sixty-five and older who ate fish at least twice a week for a period of at least six years had a 13 percent decrease in loss of cognitive functioning when compared to adults of the same age who didn't eat fish regularly. Fish is also rich in vitamin B_{12}, which helps counteract the effects of homocysteine, an amino acid that, at high levels, contributes to many diseases, including Alzheimer's disease, heart failure, and age-related macular degeneration.

essential

There is circumstantial evidence that heavy metals, like mercury, might cause or at the very least exacerbate the symptoms and progression of Alzheimer's disease. To avoid unnecessary exposure to mercury, choose low-mercury fish that are high in omega-3 fatty acids, such as salmon, tilapia, cod, and catfish.

Poultry

Poultry products, like chicken and turkey, are rich in a B vitamin called nicotinamide—or vitamin B_3—that proves promising for reversing memory loss and cognitive decline in those with Alzheimer's disease. The study that brought this information to light was an animal study published in the *Journal of Neuroscience*. Researchers genetically engineered mice to develop the equivalent of human Alzheimer's disease. Then they gave the mice an amount of vitamin B_3 that was equivalent to a human getting 2–3 grams. The mice that were treated with the vitamin supplement showed a complete reversal of symptoms, and when given a series of cognitive tests they performed as though they were never afflicted by the disease at all. The creators of the MIND diet took into account the significance of this study when determining the amount of poultry to include in the diet to provide the body with vitamin B_3.

Olive Oil

Olive oil is one of the foundations of the MIND diet. Some of the benefits of olive oil on brain health are due to its abundance of antioxidants and monounsaturated fats. Research has shown that heart-healthy unsaturated fats can protect blood vessels all over the body—including those in the brain, which in turn helps reduce the damage that can contribute to Alzheimer's disease and other forms of dementia. Other studies, however, look closely at a specific compound in olive oil called oleocanthal. Researchers have found that oleocanthal may help speed up the removal of the protein beta-amyloid, preventing it from forming the gummy plaques in the brain that are associated with Alzheimer's disease. Oleocanthal does this by increasing the production of proteins and enzymes that are necessary to carry beta-amyloid out of the brain.

Red Wine

Although excess alcohol consumption is never recommended, researchers have concluded that drinking one to two glasses of red wine per day may not only be good for heart health but may improve brain health as well. Red wine contains resveratrol—a phenolic compound that is found primarily in the skin of grapes. In preclinical studies, resveratrol has been shown to have numerous biological functions that can protect the body from neurodegenerative diseases, like Alzheimer's, as well as cancer and heart disease.

fact

A note about alcohol: Studies have shown that a moderate intake of red wine (no more than one glass per day for women or two glasses per day for men) may have protective benefits for the brain and heart. That being said, if you do not drink alcohol, it's not necessary to incorporate it into your plan to experience results.

A Note on Herbs and Spices

All herbs and spices are allowed on the MIND diet plan, and you should take advantage of them. Herbs and spices not only provide flavor to your dishes, but some of them have brain-boosting power. For example, curcumin, the active ingredient in turmeric, has been shown to reduce inflammation in the brain and help break up the plaques in the brain associated with Alzheimer's disease. Cinnamon increases the levels of compounds called neurotrophic factors in the brain. These compounds help stimulate the birth of new neurons, protect existing neurons, and protect the brain from neurodegenerative disorders. Sage helps boost memory, thyme increases the amount of DHA (an omega-3 fatty acid) in the brain, rosemary decreases cognitive decline in people with dementia, and garlic promotes better blood flow to the brain. Use caution however, as some herbs and spices are highly processed and may contain things like hydrogenated vegetable oils. Before using or purchasing a spice, look at the ingredient list to make sure that the actual spice is the only ingredient.

Suggestions for Foods to Avoid (or Limit)

The five food categories on the brain-unhealthy list are not expressly forbidden, but it's recommended to limit them or avoid them as much as possible. Those study participants who followed the MIND diet to the letter and avoided these foods had a greater success rate than those who moderately followed the diet and ate these foods in limited amounts. The recommended servings sizes for these foods if you choose to eat them are:

- Red meat—less than four servings per week
- Butter/margarine—less than 1 tablespoon per day
- Cheese—less than one serving per week
- Desserts and sweets—less than five servings per week
- Fried food and/or fast food—less than one serving per week

Think of these guidelines for the brain-unhealthy foods as upper limits. What that means is that you don't have to consume the amounts listed per day and/or week; it means that's the absolute most that you can have. For example, if you avoid red meat completely, that's great; if you decide to have red meat, you cannot exceed four servings per week.

Maintaining a Balanced Diet for Life

The MIND diet is not a fad diet or a quick weight-loss plan; it's a way of life. The people who see the most significant results from following the plan are the people who stick to the recommendations as written and follow the diet plan the longest. That being said, following the MIND diet plan doesn't mean that you'll never eat fried food or have a dessert ever again; it just means that you understand that these types of foods are a treat, and you become more mindful of how much of them you're eating and how they make you feel.

In order for a diet to become a way of life, you have to enjoy it and it has to be easy enough for you to incorporate into your lifestyle. The benefits of the MIND diet are just that: The plan is simple and consists of foods that are commonly found, easy to prepare, and taste delicious. At first, adjusting to the MIND diet may be difficult, especially if the way you eat now is different from the recommendations on the plan, but as you get into a groove, you'll find that the program is both simple and enjoyable.

CHAPTER 2

Breakfast

Hearty Whole-Grain Breakfast Bowl

With a little leftover brown rice and some quick oats, this heart-healthy meal comes together in minutes and will keep you satisfied for hours. Filled with whole-grain goodness, chopped nuts, and fruit, it's a delicious way to start any day.

Serves 1

Per Serving

Calories	343
Fat	8g
Protein	8g
Sodium	93mg
Fiber	7g
Carbohydrates	63g
Sugar	20g

¼ cup quick oats
½ cup cooked brown rice
½ cup unsweetened almond milk
1 tablespoon chopped walnuts
1 tablespoon pure maple syrup
¼ teaspoon ground cinnamon
⅛ teaspoon ground ginger
½ cup fresh blueberries

1. In a small microwave-safe bowl, add oats, rice, milk, walnuts, syrup, cinnamon, and ginger. Cover tightly with plastic wrap and microwave 3 minutes on high.
2. Carefully remove plastic wrap, stir well to combine, and top with blueberries. Serve immediately.

Oat Types

Oats come in three main types. Quick or instant oats have been precooked and dried. They have the fastest cooking time and are great for making oatmeal or adding to baked goods. Old-fashioned rolled oats have been put through a steaming process to speed up cooking. They're considered all-purpose and work well in most recipes. Steel-cut oats have a chewy texture that's good for oatmeal, but they have a longer cooking time.

Simple Vegan Pancakes

These vegan pancakes are dairy- and egg-free, which makes this dish cholesterol-free as well. But the taste and texture? It's all there! Light, fluffy, dreamy, steamy, and delicious, these pancakes are perfect. If you're watching your fat, omit the oil.

1⅓ cups white whole-wheat flour

¼ cup beet sugar

2 tablespoons ground flaxseed

1 tablespoon baking powder

6 tablespoons water

1 tablespoon vanilla extract

2 tablespoons olive oil

1⅓ cups unsweetened almond milk

1. In a medium bowl, add flour, sugar, flaxseed, and baking powder and whisk well to combine.
2. Add remaining ingredients and stir until incorporated.
3. Heat a nonstick griddle or medium skillet over medium-low to low heat. Once hot, ladle roughly ⅓ cup batter onto the hot pan. Cook until bubbles appear on the surface of pancake and the bottom is golden brown, about 2–3 minutes. Flip pancake and cook 2–3 minutes more, then remove pancake from heat. If pancakes brown too quickly, lower heat to low.
4. Repeat cooking process with remaining batter. Serve pancakes warm.

Serves 4

Per Serving

Calories	293
Fat	10g
Protein	6g
Sodium	426mg
Fiber	5g
Carbohydrates	45g
Sugar	13g

What Is Flaxseed?

Flaxseed, also known as linseed, is a healthy source of omega-3 fatty acids, fiber, and antioxidants. Ground flaxseed can be used successfully as an egg substitute in many baked goods. Simply stir 1 tablespoon ground flaxseed with 3 tablespoons water for each egg you'd like to replace, then set aside 5 minutes to thicken. Once thickened, add to the recipe as you would the egg(s).

Lemon Poppy Seed Pancakes

These pancakes are your favorite citrus muffin—but in pancake form! For the brightest flavor, use the juice and zest of 1 fresh lemon as the recipe describes, but 2 tablespoons lemon juice and ½ teaspoon lemon extract can be substituted.

Serves 4

Per Serving

Calories	256
Fat	6g
Protein	5g
Sodium	411mg
Fiber	3g
Carbohydrates	47g
Sugar	15g

Try a Ladle

Soup ladles aren't just for soup. They work wonderfully for measuring and pouring pancake batter onto any hot cooking surface. The resulting pancakes will be perfectly shaped and sized, and you'll never have to worry about messy cleanup!

¾ cup unbleached all-purpose flour
½ cup white whole-wheat flour
¼ cup granulated sugar
1 tablespoon baking powder
1 tablespoon poppy seeds
Grated zest and juice of 1 medium lemon
1 cup unsweetened almond milk
1 tablespoon agave nectar
1 tablespoon olive oil
2 teaspoons vanilla extract

1. In a medium bowl, add flours, sugar, baking powder, poppy seeds, and lemon zest and whisk together. Add lemon juice, milk, agave, oil, and vanilla and whisk until combined.
2. Heat a nonstick griddle or medium skillet over medium-low to low heat. Ladle roughly ¼ cup batter onto the hot pan. Cook until bubbles appear on the surface of pancake and the bottom is golden brown, about 2–3 minutes. Flip pancake and cook 2–3 minutes more, then remove pancake from heat. If pancakes brown too quickly, lower heat to low.
3. Repeat cooking process with remaining batter. Serve pancakes warm.

Gingerbread Pancakes

Ground ginger, cinnamon, cloves, a little brewed coffee, and brown sugar flavor these scrumptious vegan pancakes, creating a holiday-worthy breakfast you can enjoy year-round. Serve warm, drizzled with pure maple syrup.

1¼ cups white whole-wheat flour

¼ cup (packed) dark brown sugar

1 tablespoon baking powder

2 teaspoons ground ginger

1 teaspoon ground cinnamon

⅛ teaspoon ground cloves

1 cup unsweetened almond milk

¼ cup brewed coffee, cooled

2 tablespoons olive oil

2 teaspoons vanilla extract

Serves 4

Per Serving

Calories	281
Fat	9g
Protein	5g
Sodium	415mg
Fiber	5g
Carbohydrates	44g
Sugar	14g

1. In a medium bowl, add flour, sugar, baking powder, ginger, cinnamon, and cloves and whisk until all lumps are gone.
2. Add milk, coffee, oil, and vanilla and whisk well to combine.
3. Heat a nonstick griddle or medium skillet over medium-low to low heat. Ladle ¼ cup batter onto the hot pan. Cook until bubbles appear on the surface of pancake and the bottom is golden brown, about 2–3 minutes. Flip pancake and cook 2–3 minutes more, then remove pancake from heat. If pancakes brown too quickly, lower heat to low.
4. Repeat cooking process with remaining batter. Serve pancakes warm.

Peanut Butter and Jelly Pancakes

Fresh from the griddle, these vegan pancakes taste just like a warm whole-wheat peanut butter and jelly sandwich. Top the light and fluffy batter with sliced strawberries for an extra-special treat. Strawberry jam is just a suggestion; any flavor of fruit jam may be substituted instead.

Serves 4

Per Serving

Calories	295
Fat	8g
Protein	8g
Sodium	428mg
Fiber	5g
Carbohydrates	49g
Sugar	15g

Almond Milk and Other Nondairy Alternatives

The MIND diet limits the consumption of dairy products, including cow's milk, so almond milk is used throughout the recipes in this book. Its creamy, mild taste make it a great stand-in for traditional milk. Almond milk is sold in both sweetened and unsweetened forms, either plain or vanilla-flavored. An equal amount of another nondairy milk (soy, rice, coconut, hemp, or oat) may be substituted for the almond milk in any recipe in this book.

1¼ cups white whole-wheat flour

2 tablespoons granulated sugar

1 tablespoon baking powder

3 tablespoons creamy natural peanut butter

3 tablespoons strawberry jam

1¼ cups unsweetened almond milk

1 tablespoon vanilla extract

1. In a medium bowl, add flour, sugar, and baking powder and whisk well to combine.
2. Add peanut butter, jam, milk, and vanilla and stir until incorporated.
3. Heat a nonstick griddle or medium skillet over medium-low to low heat. Ladle roughly ¼ cup batter onto the hot pan. Cook until bubbles appear on the surface of pancake and the bottom is golden brown, about 2–3 minutes. Flip pancake and cook 2–3 minutes more, then remove pancake from heat. If pancakes brown too quickly, lower heat to low.
4. Repeat cooking process with remaining batter. Serve pancakes warm.

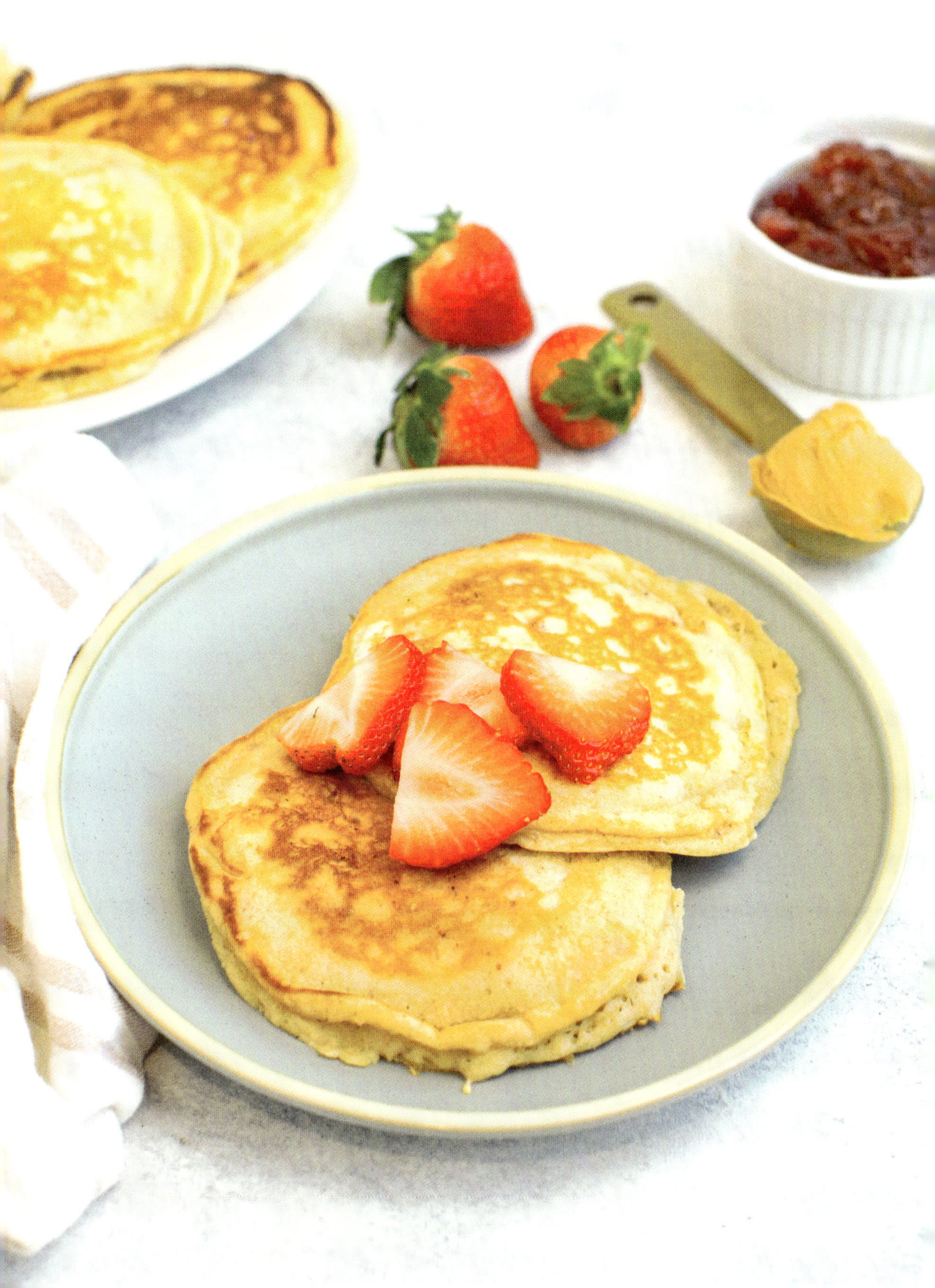

Homemade Vegan Sausage

This homemade vegan sausage is flavored with an array of herbs and has a subtle pepper kick. The recipe yields 12 (2-inch) patties, enough to feed six people. It's better tasting than commercial vegetarian sausage and much better for you too!

Serves 6

Per Serving

Calories	144
Fat	6g
Protein	4g
Sodium	76mg
Fiber	3g
Carbohydrates	19g
Sugar	1g

- 1 tablespoon ground flaxseed
- 3 tablespoons water
- 3⁄4 cup quick oats
- 2 tablespoons white whole-wheat flour
- 2 tablespoons nutritional yeast
- 1½ teaspoons ground sage
- 1½ teaspoons onion powder
- 1 teaspoon light brown sugar
- ½ teaspoon cumin seeds
- ½ teaspoon dried marjoram
- ½ teaspoon fennel seeds
- ½ teaspoon garlic powder
- ¼ teaspoon ground black pepper
- ⅛ teaspoon dried thyme
- ⅛ teaspoon ground rosemary
- 1 tablespoon low-sodium soy sauce
- 2 tablespoons olive oil, divided
- 1 cup cooked brown rice

1. In a small bowl, add flaxseed and water and stir to combine; set aside.
2. In a food processor, add oats, flour, nutritional yeast, sage, onion powder, sugar, cumin seeds, marjoram, fennel seeds, garlic powder, pepper, thyme, and rosemary and pulse well to combine.
3. Add soy sauce, 1 tablespoon oil, rice, and flaxseed mixture and pulse until the mixture gathers together in a ball.
4. Remove mixture from food processor and separate into 2-tablespoon portions. Roll into balls and press into 2" patties.
5. Heat remaining 1 tablespoon oil in a large skillet over medium-low heat. Place patties in pan and brown 2–3 minutes per side.
6. Remove patties from pan and place on a paper towel to drain. Serve immediately.

Maple Turkey Sausage

Perfect for those on the MIND diet looking for a lean breakfast meat, these homemade patties are super speedy, subtly sweet, and delicious. Feel free to substitute lean ground chicken for the turkey. For another twist on the recipe, instead of forming into patties, brown the mixture along with chopped onion, bell pepper, and garlic and serve with scrambled eggs for a hearty breakfast bowl.

2 pounds lean ground turkey

1 large egg white

1 tablespoon pure maple syrup

1 tablespoon ground sage

½ teaspoon dried red pepper flakes

½ teaspoon fennel seeds

½ teaspoon ground black pepper

½ teaspoon ground rosemary

¼ teaspoon garlic powder

1. In a large bowl, combine all ingredients and mix well using a fork or your hands. (The mixture will be sticky.) Form into 16 (2") patties.
2. Heat a nonstick griddle or medium skillet over medium heat and brown patties on both sides, about 5 minutes per side. Lower heat to medium-low or low if patties brown too quickly. Drain on paper towels, then serve.

Serves 8

Per Serving

Calories	198
Fat	9g
Protein	25g
Sodium	86mg
Fiber	0g
Carbohydrates	2g
Sugar	2g

Maple Syrup Facts

Maple syrup production begins each spring when maple trees are tapped, and their sap collected. The sap is boiled in large vats until much of the water evaporates, leaving behind a concentrated syrup that is then filtered and bottled. On average, it takes 40 gallons of sap to produce just 1 gallon of syrup! Maple syrup is extremely low in sodium, contains calcium and magnesium, and is prized for its distinctive flavor and sweetness.

Peppery Apple Chicken Sausage

A delicious change from standard ground chicken, these breakfast patties are studded with sautéed apple, onion, and garlic and have a nice peppery kick. If you prefer less spice, reduce the amount of ground pepper to ¼ teaspoon.

Serves 4

Per Serving

Calories	212
Fat	10g
Protein	21g
Sodium	67mg
Fiber	2g
Carbohydrates	9g
Sugar	6g

1 teaspoon olive oil

1 small yellow onion, peeled and chopped

2 cloves garlic, peeled and minced

1 medium apple, peeled, cored, and chopped

1 pound lean ground chicken

1 teaspoon ground sage

1 teaspoon light brown sugar

½ teaspoon ground black pepper

¼ teaspoon fennel seeds

⅛ teaspoon dried rosemary

1. Heat oil in a medium skillet over medium heat. Add onion, garlic, and apple and cook 5 minutes or until soft, stirring occasionally. Remove from heat and set aside to cool.
2. In a medium bowl, add chicken, sage, sugar, pepper, fennel seeds, and rosemary. Add cooled apple mixture and mix well with a fork or your hands. Form into 8 (3") patties.
3. Heat the same skillet over medium heat and brown patties on both sides, roughly 5 minutes per side. If patties brown too quickly, lower heat to medium-low or low. Drain on paper towels, then serve.

Two-Potato Hash Browns

In this recipe, a breakfast favorite gets a makeover—and emerges fat-free and fabulous! The prep work for this recipe is a breeze if you have a food processor with a shredder blade. If not, a standard hand grater will work just fine. If desired, sprinkle the hash browns with your choice of seasonings before serving.

2 medium potatoes, peeled and shredded

2 medium sweet potatoes, peeled and shredded

1. Place shredded potatoes in a medium stockpot and fill with water until potatoes are covered by an inch. Let rest 10 minutes.
2. Drain potatoes into a colander, rinse, and press down to remove as much water as possible.
3. Heat a medium nonstick pan or griddle over medium-low heat. Add potatoes to the hot pan. Cook 7 minutes, then flip potatoes over (this may be a bit messy) and cook 7 minutes more.
4. Remove hash browns from pan and serve immediately.

Serves 4

Per Serving

Calories	129
Fat	0g
Protein	2g
Sodium	202mg
Fiber	3g
Carbohydrates	30g
Sugar	5g

Instant Banana Oatmeal

With just three ingredients and 3 minutes of your time, this all-natural recipe is low-fat, gluten-free, cholesterol-free, free of refined sugar, high in fiber, and delicious. Enjoy as is or sprinkle with a dash of ground cinnamon.

½ cup quick oats

¾ cup water

1 medium ripe banana, peeled and mashed

1. In a small microwave-safe bowl, add oats and water and stir to combine.
2. Place bowl in microwave and cook 2 minutes on high.
3. Remove bowl from microwave and stir in the mashed banana. Serve immediately.

Serves 1

Per Serving

Calories	271
Fat	3g
Protein	7g
Sodium	10mg
Fiber	7g
Carbohydrates	55g
Sugar	15g

Instant Peaches and Cream Oatmeal

This speedy breakfast makes healthy eating enjoyable. Quick oats and canned peaches come together in minutes to create a delicious meal that'll keep you fueled all morning. The clear-plastic four-packs of 4-ounce fruit cups sold in many supermarkets are perfect for this recipe.

Serves 1

Per Serving

Calories	243
Fat	5g
Protein	7g
Sodium	149mg
Fiber	7g
Carbohydrates	44g
Sugar	14g

Eating Right on the Road

When traveling, skip the meat and eggs for breakfast and opt for oatmeal instead. This simple breakfast will keep you full without compromising your health. You can dress up plain oatmeal with fresh, dried, or canned fruit; a small packet of fruit preserves or peanut butter; or a sprinkling of brown sugar. Oatmeal contains vitamin E, iron, and calcium, and it is a good source of protein and fiber.

½ cup quick oats

¾ cup unsweetened almond milk

½ cup diced peaches in fruit juice

⅛ teaspoon ground cinnamon

1. In a small microwave-safe bowl, add oats and milk and stir to combine.
2. Place bowl in microwave and cook 2 minutes on high.
3. Remove bowl from microwave and stir in peaches with juice. Sprinkle with cinnamon. Serve immediately.

Apple, Banana, and Carrot Muffins

These muffins are packed with healthy fruit and vegetables. They must be cooled fully before serving; otherwise, they'll stick to the wrapper and resemble something more akin to a bread pudding. The muffins are best consumed the same day they're baked, but leftovers can be wrapped and frozen for freshness.

2 teaspoons ground cinnamon

7 tablespoons granulated sugar, divided

2 medium apples, peeled, cored, and chopped

1 cup grated carrot

1 medium ripe banana, peeled and mashed

¼ cup olive oil

¼ cup unsweetened almond milk

1 tablespoon vanilla extract

1¼ cups white whole-wheat flour

½ teaspoon baking powder

Serves 12

Per Serving

Calories	143
Fat	5g
Protein	2g
Sodium	30mg
Fiber	2g
Carbohydrates	24g
Sugar	12g

1. Preheat oven to 350°F. Line a 12-cup muffin pan with paper liners and set aside.
2. Make the muffin topping: In a small bowl, add cinnamon and 3 tablespoons sugar and whisk well to combine. Set aside.
3. Make the batter: In a medium bowl, add apples, carrot, and banana and stir to combine. Add oil, milk, remaining 4 tablespoons sugar, vanilla, flour, and baking powder and stir until just combined.
4. Spoon batter evenly into the muffin cups, then sprinkle cinnamon-sugar mixture evenly over batter.
5. Place pan on middle rack in oven and bake 20–25 minutes, until tester inserted into center of muffin comes out clean.
6. Remove pan from oven and place on a wire rack to cool. Cool fully, then remove muffins from pan and serve.

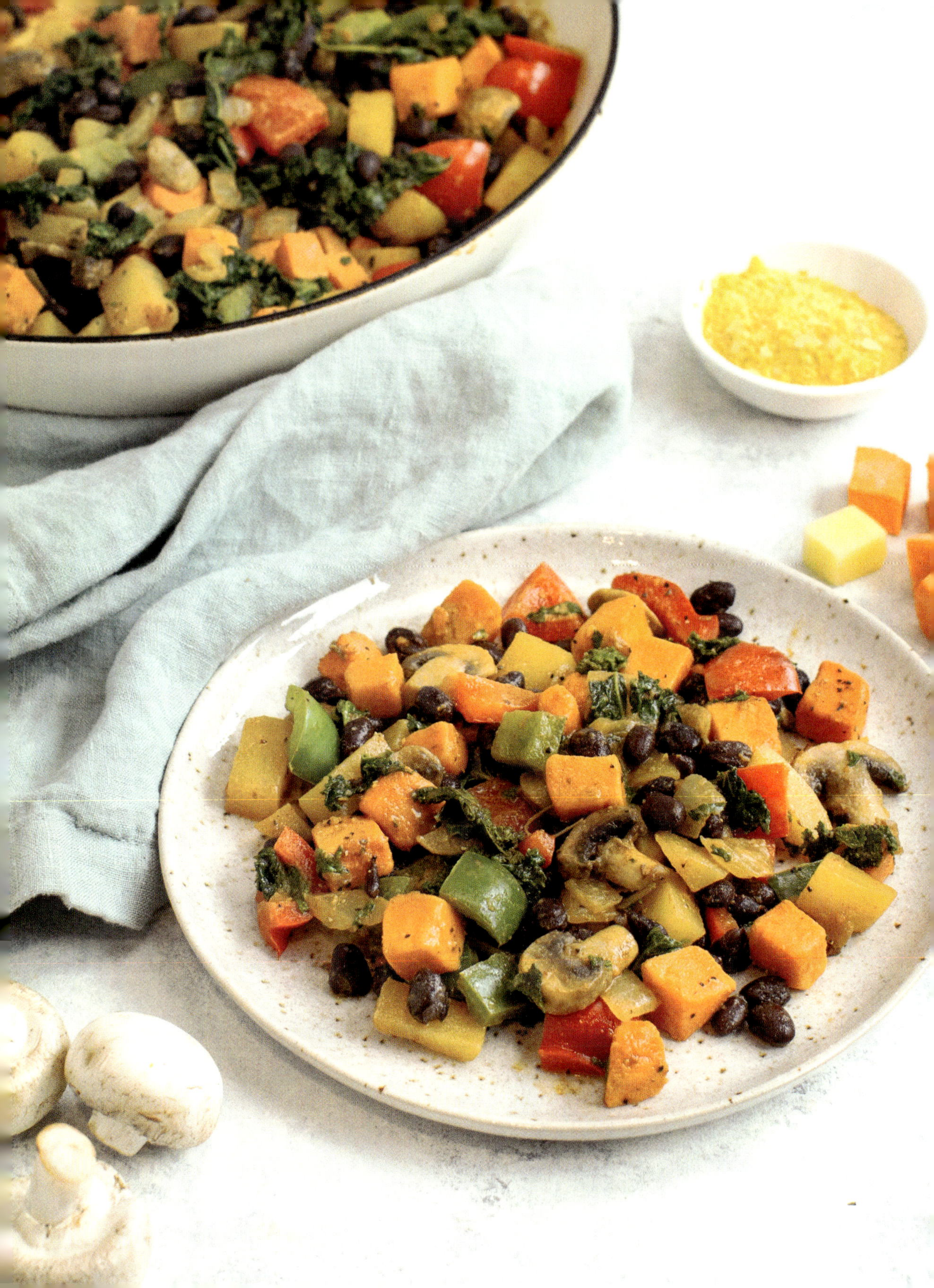

Vegetable Hash

This hearty one-pan breakfast filled with a rainbow of sautéed vegetables and beans is a great change from standard brunch fare. Be sure to cut the potatoes into a small dice so they become tender without the other vegetables overcooking. If the hash begins to stick to the pan during cooking, add a tiny bit of water or vegetable broth to the skillet and stir to release.

3 tablespoons olive oil

1 large yellow onion, peeled and diced

1 large potato, peeled and diced

1 large sweet potato, peeled and diced

3 cloves garlic, peeled and minced

1 medium green bell pepper, seeded and diced

1 medium red bell pepper, seeded and diced

8 ounces fresh mushrooms, sliced

3 cups chopped fresh kale leaves

1 (15-ounce) can black beans, drained and rinsed

2 tablespoons nutritional yeast

1 tablespoon low-sodium soy sauce

1½ teaspoons all-purpose seasoning

1 teaspoon ground paprika

1 teaspoon ground cumin

¼ teaspoon dried oregano

½ teaspoon ground black pepper

1. Heat oil in a large sauté pan over medium heat. Add onion and potatoes and cook 10 minutes, stirring often.
2. Add garlic, bell peppers, and mushrooms and cook 10 minutes, stirring often.
3. Add remaining ingredients to the pan and stir to combine. Cook and stir 5 minutes or until vegetables are tender and kale has wilted.
4. Remove from heat and serve immediately.

Serves 6

Per Serving

Calories	218
Fat	7g
Protein	9g
Sodium	602mg
Fiber	9g
Carbohydrates	32g
Sugar	6g

What Is a Hash?

Hash is a cooked dish in which all the ingredients are chopped. The word itself comes from the French verb *hacher* (meaning "to chop"). Different types of hash are popular throughout the world and most all of them combine onions and potatoes in some form, often with meat and other seasonings.

Whole-Grain Strawberry Muffins

The combination of plump, moist strawberries with the subtle crunch of cornmeal in this recipe is irresistible. Let the freshly baked muffins cool at least 10 minutes before serving to ensure the paper wrappers come off with ease.

Serves 12

Per Serving

Calories	126
Fat	4g
Protein	2g
Sodium	138mg
Fiber	2g
Carbohydrates	21g
Sugar	9g

1 cup white whole-wheat flour

½ cup cornmeal

½ cup granulated sugar

1 tablespoon baking powder

1 cup chopped fresh strawberries

1 cup unsweetened almond milk

3 tablespoons olive oil

2 teaspoons vanilla extract

1. Preheat oven to 375°F. Line a 12-cup muffin pan with paper liners and set aside.
2. In a medium bowl, add flour, cornmeal, sugar, and baking powder and whisk well to combine.
3. Add strawberries, milk, oil, and vanilla and stir until incorporated.
4. Fill muffin cups roughly two-thirds full. Place pan on middle rack in oven and bake 20 minutes, until tester inserted into center of muffin comes out clean.
5. Remove pan from oven and place on a wire rack to cool. Cool at least 10 minutes, remove muffins from pan, and serve.

Strawberry Facts

Unlike some other species of fruit, strawberries do not ripen after picking, so they must remain on the plant until peak ripeness. Strawberries are a great source of vitamin C and manganese and are believed to reduce the risk of Alzheimer's and many other ailments, including hypertension, inflammation, cancer, and cardiovascular disease.

Zucchini Muffins

This recipe is a great way to consume that bumper crop of summer zucchini. These moist muffins are delicious and freeze beautifully, so you can bake several batches to enjoy later. After shredding the zucchini, place in a clean dish towel, twist, and squeeze; you want to remove as much excess liquid as possible before making the batter.

Serves 12

Per Serving

Calories	185
Fat	8g
Protein	3g
Sodium	254mg
Fiber	2g
Carbohydrates	26g
Sugar	14g

1¼ cups shredded zucchini, drained

2 large egg whites

⅔ cup granulated sugar

⅓ cup olive oil

2 teaspoons vanilla extract

1 teaspoon ground cinnamon

¼ teaspoon ground nutmeg

2 teaspoons baking powder

1½ cups white whole-wheat flour

¼ cup chopped walnuts

¼ cup seedless raisins

1. Preheat oven to 350°F. Line a 12-cup muffin pan with paper liners and set aside.
2. In a medium bowl, add zucchini, egg whites, sugar, oil, vanilla, cinnamon, and nutmeg. Stir well.
3. Add baking powder and stir. Add flour, walnuts, and raisins and stir just until combined.
4. Divide batter evenly among muffin cups. Place pan on middle rack in oven and bake until tester inserted into center of muffin comes out clean, about 25 minutes.
5. Remove pan from oven and place on a wire rack to cool. Cool at least 10 minutes, remove muffins from pan, and serve.

Tuscan Lemon Muffins

These muffins are light and airy thanks to the ricotta cheese and are flecked with grated lemon zest with a crunch of raw sugar on top. Because of the amounts of dairy and sugar, these muffins should be an occasional treat on your MIND diet eating plan. Each moist bite is a feast for the senses, heightened by the flavor of olive oil.

Serves 12

Per Serving

Calories	189
Fat	6g
Protein	4g
Sodium	123mg
Fiber	1g
Carbohydrates	30g
Sugar	15g

Different Types of Sugar

Cane sugar comes in many varieties, including the standard white granulated sugar, brown sugar, and confectioners' sugar. But there are other alternatives. For example, beet sugar is a type of granulated sugar with vegan-friendly processing. Evaporated cane sugar, also called raw or turbinado sugar, is a natural, unrefined product that can be substituted one for one for granulated sugar. Demerara sugar is like raw sugar, but with a larger, coarser grain. It's often sprinkled on muffins before baking.

1½ cups unbleached all-purpose flour
¼ cup white whole-wheat flour
¾ cup granulated sugar
2½ teaspoons baking powder
¾ cup low-fat ricotta cheese
½ cup water
¼ cup olive oil
1 large egg
Grated zest and juice of 1 medium lemon
2 tablespoons demerara (coarse) sugar

1. Preheat oven to 375°F. Line a 12-cup muffin pan with paper liners and set aside.
2. In a large bowl, add flours, granulated sugar, and baking powder and whisk well to combine.
3. In a medium bowl, combine ricotta, water, oil, egg, and lemon zest and juice and whisk well. Add ricotta mixture to flour mixture and stir until just moist.
4. Divide batter evenly among muffin cups. Sprinkle ½ teaspoon coarse sugar over each muffin.
5. Place pan on middle rack in oven and bake 16 minutes until lightly golden.
6. Remove pan from oven and place on a wire rack to cool 5 minutes. Remove muffins from pan and serve immediately.

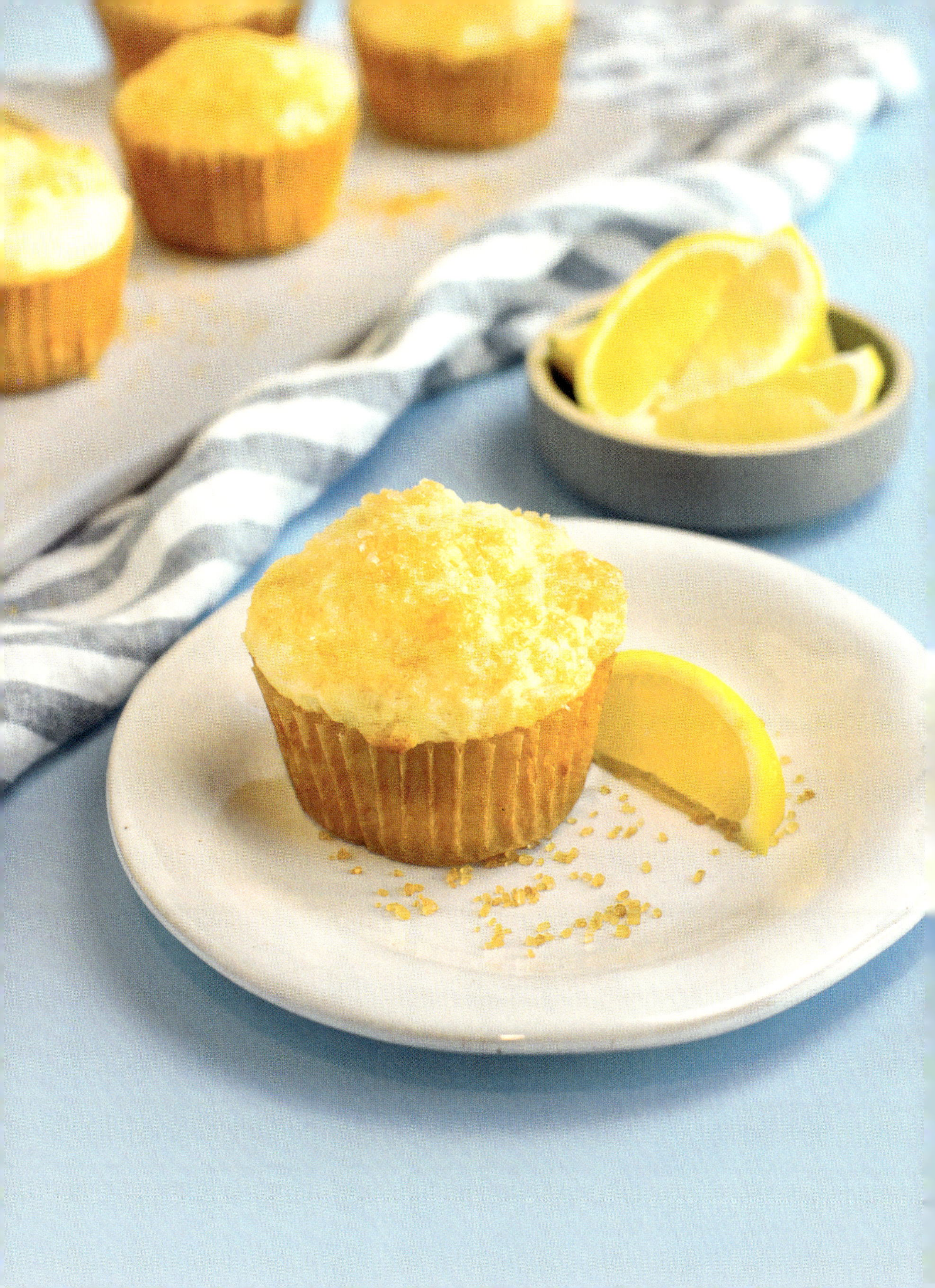

Blueberry Lemon Corn Bread

Subtly sweet and dotted with juicy blueberries, this corn bread makes a delicious breakfast or anytime treat. Either fresh or frozen berries may be used, but frozen berries must be thawed and drained before adding. If you prefer muffins, pour batter into a standard 12-cup muffin pan and bake at 400°F for 25 minutes.

Serves 16

Per Serving

Calories	161
Fat	7g
Protein	2g
Sodium	105mg
Fiber	2g
Carbohydrates	23g
Sugar	10g

Blueberry Facts

Blueberries are high in vitamins K and C as well as manganese, and they contain several antioxidants believed to inhibit memory loss, cancer, and inflammation. Fresh blueberries make an excellent addition to hot or cold cereals, baked goods, salads, and sauces, but they are perishable. To prevent spoilage, freeze blueberries and thaw as needed.

½ cup plus 1 teaspoon olive oil, divided
1 tablespoon ground flaxseed
3 tablespoons water
1 cup unsweetened almond milk
1 teaspoon lemon juice
1 cup white whole-wheat flour
1 cup cornmeal
¾ cup granulated sugar
1 tablespoon baking powder
1 teaspoon fresh-grated lemon zest
1 cup blueberries
1 teaspoon vanilla extract

1. Preheat oven to 400°F. Lightly oil an 8" square baking pan with 1 teaspoon oil and set aside.
2. In a small bowl, combine flaxseed and water and set aside. Pour milk into a measuring glass, add lemon juice, and set aside.
3. In a large bowl, add flour, cornmeal, sugar, baking powder, and lemon zest and whisk well to combine. Add blueberries to flour mixture and toss gently to coat.
4. In a small bowl, combine flaxseed mixture, milk–lemon juice mixture, remaining ½ cup oil, and vanilla and then add to flour mixture. Stir gently until just combined. Do not overmix.
5. Pour batter into prepared pan. Place pan on middle rack in oven and bake 30 minutes or until tester inserted into center comes out clean. Remove pan from oven and place on a wire rack to cool. Cool 10–15 minutes, then cut into squares and serve.

Vegan Banana Bread

This bread is irresistibly moist, tender, and bursting with banana flavor. When making banana bread, it's important not to overmix! The batter can become gummy quickly, so measure ingredients into the bowl and stir gently until just combined. This loaf can be stored in an airtight container up to 3 days.

3 tablespoons ground flaxseed

½ cup plus 1 tablespoon water

3 medium ripe bananas, peeled and mashed

1 cup granulated sugar

1½ cups white whole-wheat flour

1 tablespoon baking powder

½ cup olive oil

1 tablespoon vanilla extract

¼ cup chopped walnuts

Serves 20

Per Serving

Calories	152
Fat	7g
Protein	7g
Sodium	73mg
Fiber	2g
Carbohydrates	21g
Sugar	12g

1. Preheat oven to 350°F. Oil and flour an 8" × 3" loaf pan and set aside.
2. In a small bowl, add flaxseed and water, stir to combine, and set aside about 5 minutes to gel.
3. In a large bowl, add bananas, sugar, flour, baking powder, oil, vanilla, nuts, and flaxseed mixture. Stir gently until just combined, then transfer batter to prepared pan.
4. Place pan on middle rack in oven and bake 1 hour and 15 minutes, until tester inserted into the center comes out clean. Remove pan from oven and place on a wire rack to cool.
5. Gently invert pan to remove cooled loaf. Slice and serve.

CHAPTER 3

Appetizers and Snacks

Garlicky Steamed Clams

In this recipe, fresh clams are steamed in a simple white wine broth scented with garlic, lemon, and parsley. If you don't have a fresh lemon, substitute 2–3 generous tablespoons bottled lemon juice. Vegetable broth may be substituted for the chicken broth if desired.

Serves 4

Per Serving

Calories	99
Fat	2g
Protein	9g
Sodium	560mg
Fiber	2g
Carbohydrates	9g
Sugar	2g

Clam Facts

Although naturally higher in sodium than some other seafoods, clams can still be a part of a healthy diet. Clams are very low in fat and high in protein, iron, omega-3s, vitamin B_{12}, selenium, and manganese. Fresh uncooked clams should have a mild smell and closed shells. Any open shells should be tapped gently; clams that close can be cooked, and those that stay open are dead and should be discarded.

- 1 teaspoon olive oil
- 1 small yellow onion, peeled and chopped
- 3 cloves garlic, peeled and minced
- ¼ cup dry white wine
- 1 cup chicken broth
- Grated zest and juice of 1 medium lemon
- ¼ cup chopped fresh parsley
- ½ teaspoon ground black pepper
- 2 dozen small fresh clams, scrubbed

1. Heat oil in a large sauté pan over medium heat. Add onion and garlic and cook, stirring, 3 minutes. Add wine and stir 1 minute; then add broth, lemon zest and juice, parsley, and pepper.
2. Add clams to pan and stir well to coat. Cover pan and steam until clams open, about 7–10 minutes.
3. Uncover pan and discard any unopened clams. Serve immediately with remaining broth.

Mussels in Red Wine

Enjoy this dish as a starter for any meal or double the recipe and serve with green salad and whole-grain pasta for a spectacular main course. If you don't have fresh tomatoes and basil, substitute one 15-ounce can of no-salt-added diced tomatoes and a teaspoon of dried basil instead.

Serves 4

Per Serving

Calories	160
Fat	3g
Protein	16g
Sodium	426mg
Fiber	2g
Carbohydrates	13g
Sugar	5g

1 teaspoon olive oil

1 small yellow onion, peeled and chopped

2 cloves garlic, peeled and minced

2 medium tomatoes, chopped

¼ cup dry red wine

¾ cup vegetable juice

3 tablespoons chopped fresh basil

1 teaspoon agave nectar

¼ teaspoon dried thyme

¼ teaspoon ground black pepper

2 dozen fresh mussels, scrubbed and beards removed

1. Heat oil in a large sauté pan over medium heat. Add onion and garlic and cook, stirring, 3 minutes. Add tomatoes and cook, stirring, 2 minutes. Add wine, juice, basil, agave, thyme, and pepper.
2. Add mussels to pan and stir well to coat. Cover pan and steam until mussels open, about 5 minutes.
3. Uncover pan and discard any unopened mussels. Serve immediately with remaining broth.

Spinach and Walnut–Stuffed Mushrooms

In this dish, tender mushrooms are stuffed with a deliciously seasoned mixture of onion, garlic, walnuts, and spinach. Many supermarkets sell packaged "stuffing" mushrooms specifically for this purpose, but any good-sized fresh mushrooms will do.

Serves 8

Per Serving

Calories	58
Fat	3g
Protein	4g
Sodium	258mg
Fiber	2g
Carbohydrates	6g
Sugar	2g

16 ounces fresh stuffing mushrooms
¼ cup walnut pieces
1 small red onion, peeled and quartered
3 cloves garlic, peeled
2 cups fresh baby spinach
3 tablespoons bread crumbs
2 tablespoons nutritional yeast
1 tablespoon low-sodium soy sauce
1 teaspoon all-purpose seasoning
1 teaspoon dried basil
½ teaspoon ground black pepper
Olive oil cooking spray

1. Preheat oven to 400°F. Line a baking sheet with parchment and set aside.
2. Gently remove stems from mushrooms and set aside. Arrange mushroom caps stem side up on baking tray, allowing space between caps.
3. Place walnuts in a food processor and chop coarsely. Add mushroom stems, onion, garlic, and spinach and pulse to chop finely.
4. Transfer spinach mixture to a medium bowl. Add bread crumbs, nutritional yeast, soy sauce, seasoning, basil, and pepper and stir well to combine.
5. Fill each mushroom cap with 1–2 tablespoons filling. Spray caps lightly with cooking spray.
6. Place baking sheet on middle rack in oven and bake until tender, 35 minutes.
7. Remove from oven and serve immediately.

Shrimp with Cocktail Sauce

This dish works well with either fresh or frozen shrimp but be sure to thaw shrimp fully before serving. The cocktail sauce is spicy and tangy, almost identical to the store-bought kind, only better! When plating feel free to arrange the shrimp atop a lettuce-lined platter or hang tail-side out from stemmed glasses.

½ pound cooked medium shrimp, peeled and deveined

2½ tablespoons tomato paste

1½ tablespoons apple cider vinegar

1½ tablespoons molasses

1 tablespoon horseradish

1 teaspoon ground mustard

1 small clove garlic, peeled and grated

1. Place shrimp in a colander and rinse well under cold water. Plate shrimp, cover, and refrigerate until serving.
2. In a small bowl, add tomato paste, vinegar, molasses, horseradish, mustard, and garlic and stir to combine. Cover and refrigerate at least 1 hour, then serve.

Serves 4

Per Serving

Calories	106
Fat	1g
Protein	14g
Sodium	618mg
Fiber	1g
Carbohydrates	10g
Sugar	7g

Shrimp Facts

Shrimp are low in calories, high in protein, and contain many key nutrients, including selenium, vitamin B_{12}, phosphorous, choline, copper, and iodine. Shrimp even contain antioxidants—something rarely found in meat. Shrimp are high in cholesterol but contain very little saturated fat, making them a healthy part of a MIND diet when eaten in moderation.

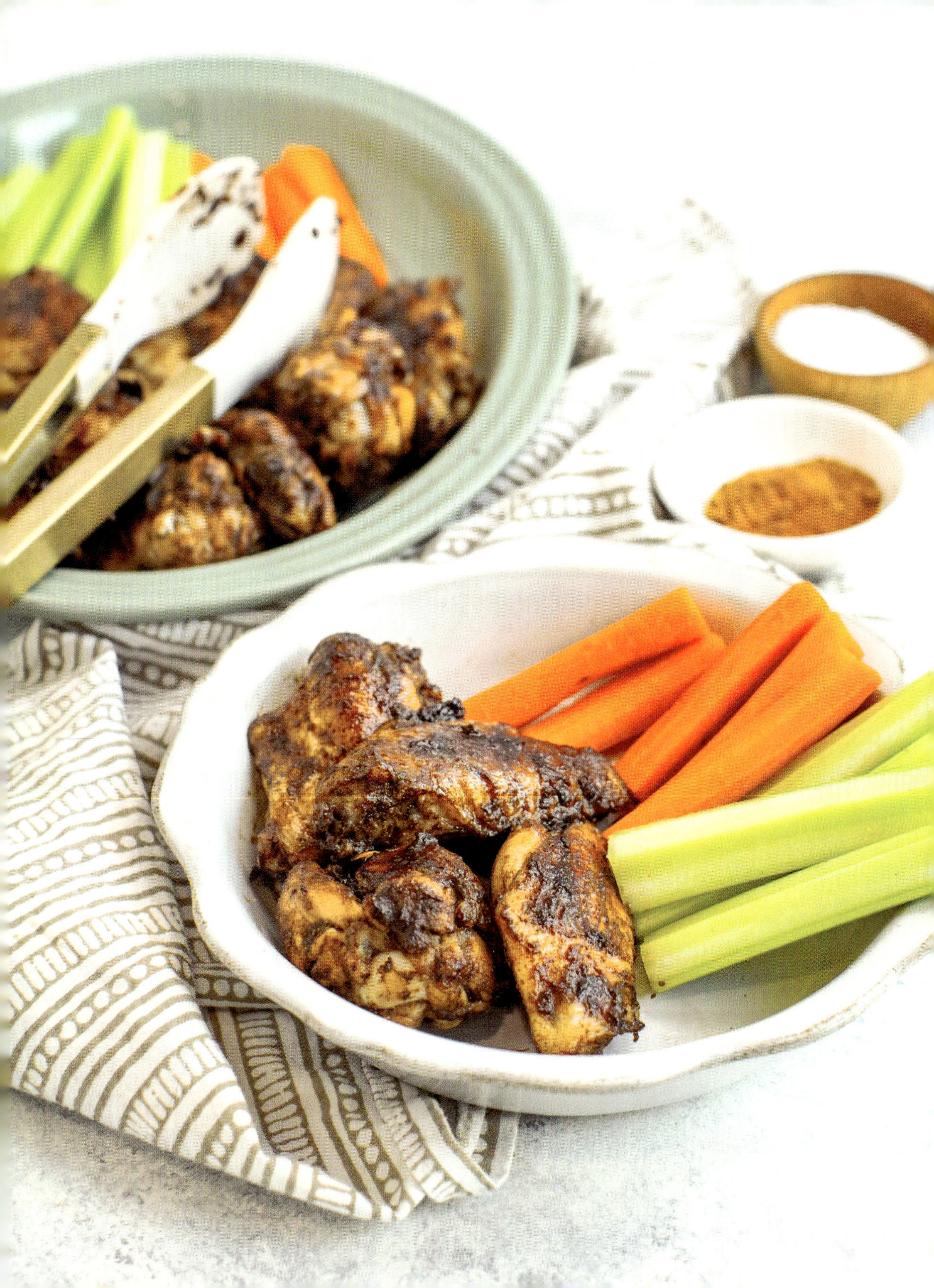

Glazed Balsamic Chicken Wings

Chicken wings are a consummate party food. Here's a less guilty way of satisfying that indulgence. This recipe produces deliciously sticky wings with a crispy, caramelized coating.

3 pounds chicken wings, wing tips removed

½ cup red currant jelly

⅓ cup balsamic vinegar

1 teaspoon low-sodium soy sauce

1 teaspoon ground cayenne

1 teaspoon garlic powder

1 teaspoon onion powder

Serves 6

Per Serving

Calories	513
Fat	27g
Protein	40g
Sodium	198mg
Fiber	0g
Carbohydrates	22g
Sugar	15g

1. Preheat oven to 450°F. Line a baking sheet with aluminum foil and set aside.
2. Place wings in a large bowl and set aside.
3. In a small saucepan over medium-high heat, add jelly, vinegar, and soy sauce. Bring mixture to a boil, stirring occasionally. Boil 5–7 minutes until mixture turns thick and glossy.
4. While mixture is boiling, place cayenne, garlic powder, and onion powder in a small bowl. Whisk well to combine.
5. Remove thickened jelly mixture from heat and whisk in seasoning mixture. Pour mixture over wings and toss well to coat.
6. Using tongs, remove coated wings from bowl and arrange on the baking sheet meaty-side down. Place sheet on middle rack in oven and bake 10–12 minutes. Flip wings, then return to oven and bake another 10–12 minutes until cooked through.
7. Transfer remaining sauce in the bowl to a small saucepan, place over medium-high heat, and bring to a boil. Reduce heat to low and simmer 1–2 minutes, stirring occasionally.
8. At the end of the baking time, turn on the broiler and broil wings 3–4 minutes more until chicken is richly colored and glossy. Remove from oven and drizzle remaining sauce over wings. Serve immediately.

Citrus-Marinated Shrimp Cocktail

A delightful change from classic shrimp cocktail, this refreshing appetizer will leave you wanting more. Either fresh or thawed frozen shrimp may be used. Garnish with citrus wedges and fresh cilantro when serving.

Serves 4

Per Serving

Calories	72
Fat	1g
Protein	13g
Sodium	550mg
Fiber	0g
Carbohydrates	2g
Sugar	1g

½ pound cooked medium shrimp, peeled and deveined

⅓ cup orange juice

⅓ cup lemon juice

¼ cup ketchup

1 tablespoon olive oil

1 medium shallot, peeled and minced

1½ teaspoons horseradish

2 tablespoons chopped fresh cilantro

1. In a large bowl, combine all ingredients and mix well. Cover and refrigerate 3–6 hours.
2. Drain and serve.

Frozen Shrimp

Much of the "fresh" shrimp sold in supermarkets has been previously frozen and thawed, so don't be discouraged from buying the prepackaged kind. To thaw frozen shrimp, place in a colander in the sink and run under cold water for about 5 minutes, tossing periodically to ensure all are defrosting. Test the shrimp by bending gently; once thawed, they will be soft and pliable.

Pan-Fried Calamari

If you love deep-fried calamari, try this healthier homemade version. Fresh or frozen squid is sold in many supermarkets and often comes pretrimmed and cleaned. When cooking, be sure to watch the clock carefully; calamari becomes rubbery if left in the oil for too long.

Serves 4

Per Serving

Calories	73
Fat	4g
Protein	5g
Sodium	12mg
Fiber	0g
Carbohydrates	4g
Sugar	0g

3 tablespoons white whole-wheat flour

1 tablespoon cornmeal

4 large squid tubes (about 4 ounces), washed and sliced into ¼"-thick rings

Olive oil for frying

Juice of 1 medium lemon

1. In a large zip-top bag, add flour and cornmeal. Seal and shake well to combine. Add squid, seal the bag, and shake well to coat.
2. Place a large skillet over medium heat. Add enough oil to reach a depth of 2".
3. Loop some floured rings over the handle of a wooden spoon until you have a good batch for frying; add rings to oil one by one in a clockwise fashion until pan is full. Keep an eye on the time—at the 2½-minute-mark, remove rings in clockwise order from your starting point in the pan.
4. Place cooked calamari on a plate lined with paper towels to drain until all squid has been cooked. Repeat process with remaining calamari until all are cooked.
5. Sprinkle calamari with lemon juice and serve immediately.

Cilantro Lime Black Bean Spread

This bean spread is made up of black beans, fresh cilantro, and garlic with a zippy lime kick. Spread in sandwiches or serve with fresh vegetables and tortilla chips.

Yields 1½ cups

Per Serving (Serving size: ¼ cup)

Calories	68
Fat	0g
Protein	4g
Sodium	163mg
Fiber	5g
Carbohydrates	13g
Sugar	0g

1 (15-ounce) can black beans, drained and rinsed

¼ cup fresh cilantro

2 cloves garlic, peeled

Juice of 1 medium lime

1½ teaspoons ground cumin

½ teaspoon ground coriander

¼ teaspoon chili seasoning

¼ teaspoon ground black pepper

⅛ teaspoon ground cayenne

Place all ingredients in a food processor and pulse until smooth. Serve immediately or cover and refrigerate until serving.

Baked Tofu with Tangy Dipping Sauce

This recipe will make a tofu lover out of you! To prepare you will want to press your drained tofu between paper towels for 30 minutes per side.

Olive oil cooking spray
1 pound extra-firm tofu, drained and pressed for 1 hour
1 large egg white
1 tablespoon water
½ cup bread crumbs
1 tablespoon dried parsley
1 teaspoon dried Italian seasoning
1 teaspoon ground paprika
1 teaspoon onion powder
½ teaspoon garlic powder
½ teaspoon ground black pepper
1 (8-ounce) can tomato sauce
1 tablespoon apple cider vinegar
1 tablespoon molasses
1 tablespoon honey
1 tablespoon ground mustard
½ teaspoon ground cumin
⅛ teaspoon ground cayenne

1. Preheat oven to 425°F. Spray a baking sheet lightly with olive oil cooking spray and set aside.
2. Slice your pressed tofu in half lengthwise, then slice each half into 8 equal pieces.
3. In a medium shallow bowl, beat egg white and water together until slightly foamy.
4. In another medium bowl, add bread crumbs, parsley, Italian seasoning, paprika, onion powder, garlic powder, and pepper and whisk well to combine.
5. Dip each piece of tofu in egg white, then press into the bread crumbs to coat. Place coated tofu cutlets on prepared baking sheet.
6. Place baking sheet on middle rack in oven and bake 10 minutes. Remove from oven, gently flip, and return to oven to bake another 10 minutes.
7. While tofu is baking, in a small saucepan add tomato sauce, vinegar, molasses, honey, mustard, cumin, and cayenne. Heat over medium-low heat and stir frequently until mixture begins to bubble, about 3–5 minutes. Remove from heat and pour into a small serving bowl.
8. Remove tofu from oven and serve immediately with prepared sauce.

Serves 8

Per Serving

Calories	124
Fat	4g
Protein	8g
Sodium	156mg
Fiber	2g
Carbohydrates	15g
Sugar	8g

Versatile Tofu

Tofu soaks up flavors like nothing else and can be added to almost any type of dish, providing added protein, calcium, and iron. Cube a pound of tofu, add to assorted vegetables, and roast. Slice into sticks, toss with a little nutritional yeast, and bake. Crumble and add to a vegetable stir-fry with brown rice. Or use instead of chicken in a vegetarian noodle soup.

Lemony Herbed Chicken Wings

This recipe is flavored with a little olive oil, some rosemary, garlic, and the secret ingredient—lemon juice. This citrusy marinade imbues the chicken with moist flavor and the most delectable aroma. Allow the chicken to rest in the marinade as long as possible, preferably overnight.

Serves 8

Per Serving

Calories	496
Fat	34g
Protein	41g
Sodium	167mg
Fiber	0g
Carbohydrates	1g
Sugar	0g

4 pounds chicken wings, wing tips removed

⅓ cup lemon juice

⅓ cup olive oil

1 tablespoon dried rosemary, crushed

4 cloves garlic, peeled and minced

½ teaspoon ground black pepper

1. Arrange chicken wings in an oven-safe baking dish without crowding (if necessary, use two dishes). Set aside.
2. In a small bowl, add lemon juice, oil, rosemary, garlic, and pepper and whisk well to combine. Pour over chicken wings and turn to coat.
3. Cover the dish and refrigerate as long as possible, preferably 8 hours or even overnight. Turn wings at least once while marinating.
4. When ready to cook, preheat oven to 400°F. Place wings in uncovered dish on middle rack in oven and bake until golden and crisp, 30–60 minutes depending upon the size of wings. The internal temperature should reach 165°F and the juices should run clear. Remove from oven and let cool.
5. Serve warm or at room temperature. Wings can also be refrigerated for later consumption and served cold.

Don't Waste Those Bones

Animal bones can't be composted, but they can be used to flavor recipes, especially homemade broth. Place bones and other scraps in a stockpot, add water to cover, and bring to a boil over high heat. Once boiling, reduce heat to low, cover, and simmer an hour or more. Strain and then discard the spent bones.

Roasted Chickpeas

Roasted chickpeas make a delicious snack, especially when they're eaten straight out of the oven. Serve them as a warm appetizer in a bowl, just as you would nuts, or toss them with salads instead of croutons. They're totally addictive, so watch out—you may find yourself eating more than just the ¼-cup serving!

1 teaspoon plus 1 tablespoon olive oil, divided

2 (15-ounce) cans chickpeas, drained, rinsed, and patted dry

1 teaspoon all-purpose seasoning

½ teaspoon ground black pepper

1. Preheat oven to 400°F. Lightly oil a medium cast iron skillet or baking sheet with 1 teaspoon oil and set aside.
2. In a medium bowl, add remaining 1 tablespoon oil, chickpeas, seasoning, and pepper and toss well to coat.
3. Transfer chickpeas to skillet or baking sheet and spread evenly. Place on middle rack in oven and bake 10 minutes. Stir chickpeas and bake another 10 minutes. Stir one more time and bake a final 10 minutes.
4. Remove from oven and serve immediately.

Serves 8

Per Serving

Calories	95
Fat	2g
Protein	4g
Sodium	309mg
Fiber	4g
Carbohydrates	15g
Sugar	3g

Green Pea "Guacamole"

Chunky, flavorful, and totally satisfying, this dip has all the amazing taste of traditional avocado guacamole. Bonus? It's gorgeous green color doesn't fade or turn brown, even after days in the refrigerator. Serve with chips or dollop over nachos, tacos, burritos, and more.

Yields 2½ cups

Per Serving (Serving size: ¼ cup)

Calories	43
Fat	1g
Protein	2g
Sodium	36mg
Fiber	2g
Carbohydrates	6g
Sugar	2g

2½ cups frozen green peas

¼ cup water

1 small red onion, peeled and quartered

1 small jalapeño pepper, seeded (if desired) and quartered

1 small tomato, quartered

1 tablespoon chopped fresh cilantro

1 clove garlic, peeled

1 tablespoon lime juice

1 tablespoon olive oil

¼ teaspoon ground coriander

¼ teaspoon ground cumin

½ teaspoon ground black pepper

1. Place peas and water in a medium microwave-safe bowl, cover with plastic wrap, and microwave 5 minutes on high. Drain and place in a food processor. Pulse to chop coarsely.
2. Add remaining ingredients to food processor; cover and pulse to combine.
3. Cover and refrigerate until serving.

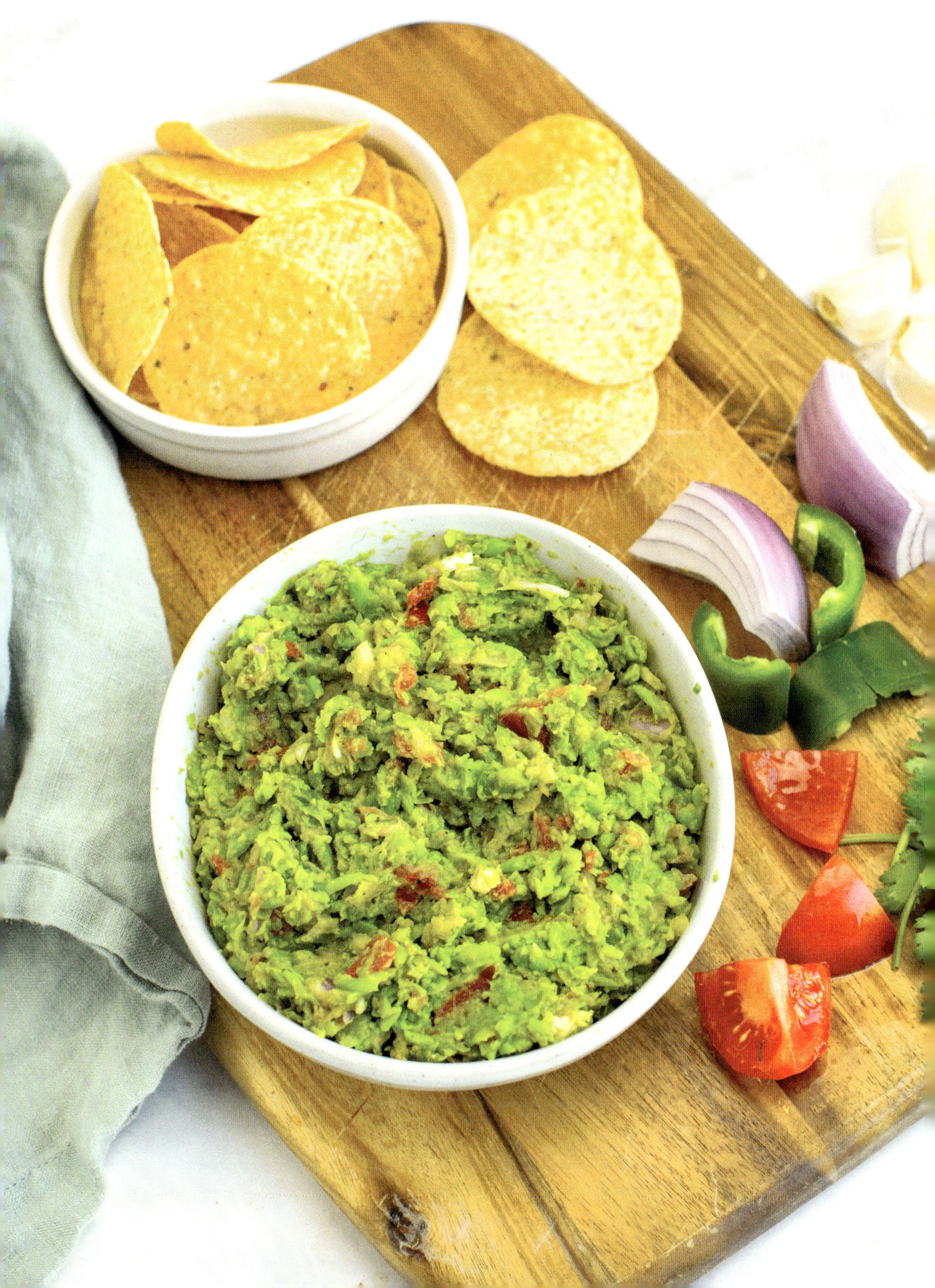

Sweet Clementine Salsa

As colorful as it is tangy, this bright orange salsa is bursting with citrus. Easy-peel clementines make preparation a snap, but feel free to substitute another citrus fruit in the off-season. Pulse minimally in your food processor for an extra-chunky salsa to enjoy with chips, or purée for a fat-free drizzle to use over salads, grilled meat, and more.

Yields 1½ cups

Per Serving (Serving size: ¼ cup)

Calories	33
Fat	0g
Protein	1g
Sodium	3mg
Fiber	1g
Carbohydrates	8g
Sugar	6g

Clementine Facts

A cross between a Chinese mandarin and a conventional orange, clementines are slightly sweeter than an orange, but lower in sugar. Clementines are low in calories and high in vitamin C, potassium, beta-carotene, and fiber. Look for them beginning in the fall; their peak season stretches into the new year.

4 small clementines, peeled
1 small red onion, peeled and quartered
2 cloves garlic, peeled
½ medium orange bell pepper, seeded and quartered
1 tablespoon fresh cilantro
1 tablespoon orange juice
1 teaspoon apple cider vinegar
¼ teaspoon ground cumin
⅛ teaspoon dried red pepper flakes
⅛ teaspoon chili seasoning

Place all ingredients in a food processor and pulse to combine. Cover and refrigerate until serving.

Curried Potato Croquettes

This recipe yields twenty-four croquettes, enough to serve twelve people as an appetizer or eight as a main course. Serve with chutney or ketchup.

- 3 teaspoons olive oil, divided
- 6 medium potatoes, peeled and diced
- 2 tablespoons nutritional yeast
- 2 teaspoons ground cumin
- 2 teaspoons curry powder
- 1½ teaspoons garlic powder
- 1 teaspoon light brown sugar
- 1 teaspoon cumin seeds
- ¾ teaspoon dried oregano
- ½ teaspoon ground coriander
- ¼ teaspoon ground cayenne
- ¼ teaspoon ground ginger
- 1 tablespoon low-sodium soy sauce
- 2 tablespoons chopped fresh cilantro
- ¾ cup bread crumbs

1. Preheat oven to 400°F. Use 1 teaspoon oil to lightly oil two baking sheets and set aside.
2. Place potatoes in a medium stockpot and add enough water to cover by 1"–2". Bring to a boil over high heat, then reduce heat to medium and boil 20 minutes.
3. Meanwhile, in a small bowl, add nutritional yeast, ground cumin, curry powder, garlic powder, sugar, cumin seeds, oregano, coriander, cayenne, and ginger and whisk well to combine.
4. Drain potatoes, then mash. Add seasoning mixture, soy sauce, remaining 2 teaspoons oil, and cilantro and stir to combine.
5. Place bread crumbs in a medium shallow bowl.
6. To form croquettes, scoop roughly 2 tablespoons potato mixture, roll into a ball, and flatten into a 2"–3" patty. Press potato cake into bread crumbs, then gently flip to coat second side. Place breaded croquette on the baking sheet and repeat with remaining ingredients until you have 24 croquettes.
7. Place baking sheets on middle rack in oven and bake 12–15 minutes until golden brown on the bottom. Gently flip, return to oven, and bake another 12–15 minutes until golden brown.
8. Remove from oven and serve immediately.

Serves 12

Per Serving

Calories	118
Fat	2g
Protein	3g
Sodium	92mg
Fiber	2g
Carbohydrates	23g
Sugar	2g

Preserving Dried Herbs and Spices

Many people position their spice rack close to the stove for easy access during cooking. But the proximity of the heat and humidity compromises flavor. To maximize freshness, store dried herbs and seasonings in a cool, dark cabinet away from direct sunlight and cooking.

Basil Pesto Hummus

This scrumptious hummus is light and fluffy and flavored with the fresh taste of basil. It's also a nutritional powerhouse, high in vitamins (A, C, and K), folic acid, antioxidants, protein, and fiber. Serve with tortilla chips and fresh vegetables. Baby spinach may be substituted for the fresh arugula if desired.

Yields 2 cups

Per Serving (Serving size: 1⁄4 cup)

Calories	108
Fat	6g
Protein	5g
Sodium	213mg
Fiber	3g
Carbohydrates	10g
Sugar	0g

1⁄4 cup walnut pieces

1⁄3 cup fresh basil

1⁄3 cup fresh arugula

4 cloves garlic, peeled and minced

3 tablespoons nutritional yeast

1 tablespoon lemon juice

1 tablespoon low-sodium soy sauce

1 tablespoon olive oil

1 tablespoon tahini

1⁄2 teaspoon ground black pepper

1 (15-ounce) can chickpeas, drained and liquid reserved

1. Place walnuts in a food processor and pulse until chopped.
2. Add basil, arugula, garlic, nutritional yeast, lemon juice, soy sauce, oil, tahini, pepper, chickpeas, and 1⁄4 cup reserved chickpea liquid and pulse until smooth.
3. Serve immediately or cover and refrigerate until serving.

Crisp and Crunchy Kale Popcorn

If you like kale chips, you're going to love this yummy snack. The flavored popcorn and crackly kale come together in a crisp and crunchy marriage of tastes and textures. It's a deliciously healthy, fun, and filling way to satisfy your between-meal cravings.

- 8 cups chopped fresh kale leaves
- 2 tablespoons nutritional yeast, divided
- 1½ teaspoons garlic powder, divided
- ½ teaspoon low-sodium soy sauce
- ½ teaspoon olive oil
- 1 teaspoon sriracha
- 8 cups air-popped popcorn
- ½ teaspoon ground cumin
- ½ teaspoon ground paprika
- ¼ teaspoon dried oregano
- ¼ teaspoon dried thyme
- ⅛ teaspoon ground cayenne
- Olive oil cooking spray

Serves 10

Per Serving

Calories	38
Fat	1g
Protein	2g
Sodium	23mg
Fiber	2g
Carbohydrates	7g
Sugar	0g

1. Preheat oven to 300°F. Line two baking sheets with parchment and set aside.
2. Place kale in a large bowl.
3. In a small bowl, add 1 tablespoon nutritional yeast, ½ teaspoon garlic powder, soy sauce, oil, and sriracha and stir well to combine. Drizzle mixture over kale and toss 1–2 minutes using your hands to coat.
4. Spread kale evenly on baking sheets so the pieces have space between them. Place on middle rack in oven and bake 10 minutes. Stir gently, then bake another 3 minutes until kale is dark and crisp. Remove from oven and set aside.
5. Place popcorn in a large bowl. In a small bowl, add cumin, paprika, oregano, thyme, cayenne, and remaining garlic powder and nutritional yeast and stir to combine. Spray popcorn lightly with cooking spray, sprinkle with seasoning mix, and toss well to coat. Spread popcorn evenly on a parchment-lined baking sheet. Place on middle rack in oven and bake 5 minutes until mixture is lightly toasted.
6. Remove popcorn from oven and transfer to a large bowl. Add kale chips and toss gently to combine. Divide mixture evenly between two parchment-lined baking sheets, return to middle rack in oven, and bake another 3–5 minutes until toasted.
7. Remove from oven and place on a wire rack to cool. Serve warm or cool.

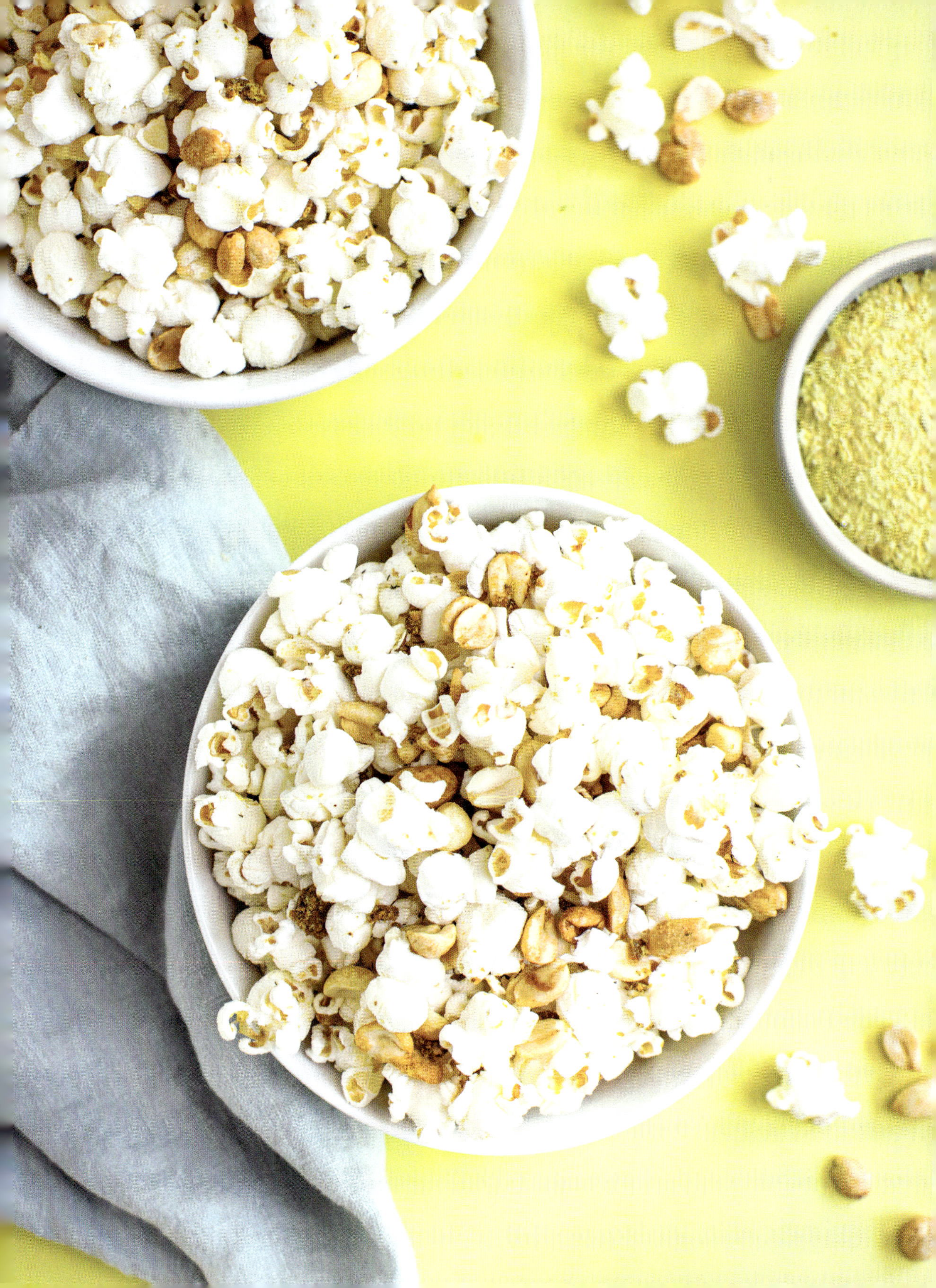

Party Mix Popcorn

An addictively crunchy alternative to potato chips and other salty snacks, this deliciously seasoned party mix will make a MIND diet snack lover out of you. For variety, substitute 2 cups of pretzels or bite-sized shredded wheat cereal for an equal amount of the popcorn.

Serves 10

Per Serving

Calories	121
Fat	7g
Protein	5g
Sodium	51mg
Fiber	3g
Carbohydrates	10g
Sugar	1g

10 cups air-popped popcorn

1 cup unsalted peanuts

2 tablespoons nutritional yeast

1 tablespoon low-sodium soy sauce

1 teaspoon garlic powder

½ teaspoon onion powder

½ teaspoon lemon-pepper seasoning

¼ teaspoon dried dill

⅛ teaspoon ground mustard

Olive oil cooking spray

1. Preheat oven to 300°F. Line two baking sheets with parchment and set aside.
2. Place popcorn and peanuts in a large bowl.
3. In a small bowl, add nutritional yeast, soy sauce, garlic powder, onion powder, lemon-pepper, dill, and mustard and whisk well to combine. Spray popcorn mixture with oil, add seasoning blend, and toss well to coat; spray with a little more oil as necessary to get the seasoning to stick.
4. Spread party mix evenly on the prepared baking sheets. Lightly spray again with oil. Place sheets on middle rack in oven and bake 5 minutes. Stir mix, rotate sheets, and bake another 4–5 minutes, until lightly toasted.
5. Remove from oven and place on a wire rack to cool. Serve warm or cool.

Cinnamon-Sweet Cracker Jack Popcorn

This popcorn tastes like homemade Cracker Jack, but with very little sugar and zero salt. It has the perfect hint of sugar and spice and couldn't be easier to make. If you're feeling extra hungry, add ¼ cup of unsalted roasted peanuts, double the batch, and dig in!

Serves 4

Per Serving

Calories	42
Fat	0g
Protein	1g
Sodium	0mg
Fiber	1g
Carbohydrates	9g
Sugar	3g

1 tablespoon granulated sugar

⅛ teaspoon ground cinnamon

4 cups air-popped popcorn

Olive oil cooking spray

1. Preheat oven to 300°F. Line a baking sheet with parchment and set aside.
2. In a small bowl, add sugar and cinnamon and whisk well to combine. Place popcorn in a large bowl and spray with oil, then add cinnamon-sugar and toss well to coat.
3. Spread popcorn evenly on the baking sheet. Lightly spray again with oil and sprinkle with any residual seasoning. Place sheet on middle rack in oven and bake 4–5 minutes. Stir mix, rotate sheet, and bake another 4–5 minutes, until lightly golden.
4. Remove from oven and place on a wire rack to cool. Serve warm or cool.

CHAPTER 4

Soups and Salads

Slow Cooker Lentil Vegetable Soup

This tomato-rich, thick, and delicious soup isn't just healthy and satisfying. Thanks to the slow cooker, it's also convenient, making it that much easier to stay true to your diet. This recipe calls for fresh baby spinach, but you can substitute an equal amount of frozen spinach if you prefer.

Serves 8

Per Serving

Calories	163
Fat	0g
Protein	9g
Sodium	751mg
Fiber	6g
Carbohydrates	32g
Sugar	8g

1 large yellow onion, peeled and diced
3 medium carrots, peeled and diced
2 medium stalks celery, trimmed and diced
3 cloves garlic, peeled and minced
1 cup uncooked lentils, rinsed
1 cup fresh or frozen corn kernels
10 ounces fresh baby spinach
1 (14.5-ounce) can no-salt-added diced tomatoes, with juice
3 cups vegetable broth
3 cups vegetable juice
2 cups water
1 tablespoon low-sodium soy sauce
1 teaspoon all-purpose seasoning
1 teaspoon dried basil
½ teaspoon dried thyme
½ teaspoon ground black pepper

1. Place all ingredients in a slow cooker and stir well to combine. It may be a bit crowded initially because of spinach but will quickly cook down.
2. Cover the slow cooker and cook on low 6–8 hours or on high 4–5 hours, stirring occasionally if possible. Cook until vegetables and lentils are tender. Serve hot.

Vegetable Potpie Stew

This crustless potpie is the perfect go-to comfort meal. A traditional combination of vegetables simmered in a creamy, herb-flavored broth, it's best served over cooked brown rice or eggless noodles or partnered with toasted bread or biscuits.

- 1 cup unsweetened almond milk
- 3 tablespoons white whole-wheat flour
- 2 cups vegetable broth
- 3 tablespoons nutritional yeast
- 1 tablespoon low-sodium soy sauce
- 2 teaspoons all-purpose seasoning
- ½ teaspoon dried thyme
- ½ teaspoon ground mustard
- ½ teaspoon ground sage
- ¼ teaspoon dried dill
- 1 teaspoon olive oil
- 1 medium yellow onion, peeled and diced
- 4 cloves garlic, peeled and minced
- 3 medium carrots, peeled and diced
- 3 medium stalks celery, trimmed and diced
- 2 cups diced fresh mushrooms
- 1 cup frozen green peas
- 1 cup frozen corn kernels
- 1 cup fresh or frozen green beans, cut into 1" pieces
- 1 pound red potatoes, diced
- 2 cups chopped fresh baby spinach
- 1 (15-ounce) can chickpeas, drained and rinsed
- ½ teaspoon ground black pepper

Serves 8

Per Serving

Calories	180
Fat	2g
Protein	8g
Sodium	757mg
Fiber	7g
Carbohydrates	34g
Sugar	7g

1. In a medium bowl, add milk and flour and whisk until smooth. Add broth, nutritional yeast, soy sauce, seasoning, thyme, mustard, sage, and dill and whisk well until combined. Set aside.
2. Heat oil in a large stockpot over medium heat. Add onion and cook, stirring, 2 minutes, until it begins to sweat. Add garlic, carrots, celery, and mushrooms and sauté 5 minutes, until mushrooms begin to release their juice.
3. Add peas, corn, green beans, potatoes, spinach, and chickpeas and stir to combine. Pour liquid mixture over vegetables and stir to coat. Bring mixture to a boil over high heat, then lower heat, cover, and simmer until vegetables are tender, about 20 minutes.
4. Remove from heat. Season with pepper. Serve hot.

Slow Cooker Sweet Potato and Kale Stew

Chock-full of the good stuff—vitamins, antioxidants, iron, calcium, fiber, and more—and with the most stupendous combination of flavors, this hearty, MIND diet-approved stew will leave you feeling fantastic. Serve over cooked brown rice for a complete meal.

Serves 8

Per Serving

Calories	179
Fat	3g
Protein	6g
Sodium	870mg
Fiber	7g
Carbohydrates	31g
Sugar	10g

3 medium sweet potatoes, peeled and cubed
1 large yellow onion, peeled and diced
3 medium carrots, peeled and sliced
5 cloves garlic, peeled and minced
1 medium red bell pepper, seeded and diced
8 cups chopped fresh kale leaves
1 (14.5-ounce) can no-salt-added diced tomatoes, with juice
1 (15-ounce) can kidney beans, drained and rinsed
4 cups vegetable broth
1 (13.5-ounce) can light coconut milk
2 tablespoons tomato paste
1 tablespoon agave nectar
1 tablespoon apple cider vinegar
1 tablespoon lime juice
1 tablespoon Thai red curry paste
1 tablespoon ground cumin
1 teaspoon ground paprika
1½ teaspoons all-purpose seasoning
1 teaspoon ground coriander
½ teaspoon dried oregano
¼ teaspoon dried thyme
½ teaspoon ground black pepper

1. Place all ingredients in a slow cooker and carefully stir to combine (it will be quite full).
2. Cover slow cooker, set to high, and cook 6 hours, stirring occasionally if possible. Serve hot.

Hearty Slow Cooker Black Bean Soup

This recipe gives you a slow-cooked soup that will fill your house with the most spectacular aroma. For less spice, seed the jalapeño before mincing. And remember, don't drain the beans! The liquid becomes part of the stock.

1 medium yellow onion, peeled and diced
3 cloves garlic, peeled
2 medium stalks celery, trimmed and diced
1 medium green bell pepper, seeded and diced
1 medium red bell pepper, seeded and diced
1 medium jalapeño pepper, minced
1 (14.5-ounce) can no-salt-added diced tomatoes, with juice
3 (15-ounce) cans black beans, undrained
5 cups vegetable broth
⅓ cup red wine
1 tablespoon apple cider vinegar
1 tablespoon agave nectar
1 bay leaf
1 tablespoon ground cumin
2 teaspoons all-purpose seasoning
2 teaspoons ground paprika
1½ teaspoons dried oregano
1 teaspoon ground coriander
½ teaspoon dried thyme
¼ teaspoon dried red pepper flakes
½ teaspoon ground black pepper

Serves 6

Per Serving

Calories	251
Fat	1g
Protein	14g
Sodium	972mg
Fiber	17g
Carbohydrates	46g
Sugar	6g

1. Place all ingredients in a slow cooker and stir well to combine. Cover, set to low, and cook 7 hours, or set to high and cook 5 hours, stirring occasionally if possible.
2. Before serving, remove bay leaf and discard. Transfer roughly a third of the soup to a food processor and purée. Return soup to slow cooker and stir to combine. Serve hot.

Pumpkin Ginger Soup

This Pumpkin Ginger Soup is a vibrant and flavorful dish whose subtle sweetness adds sophistication to any meal, especially holiday celebrations. If you don't have fresh ginger, substitute ¾ teaspoon ground ginger.

Serves 4

Per Serving

Calories	158
Fat	6g
Protein	3g
Sodium	861mg
Fiber	6g
Carbohydrates	24g
Sugar	13g

1 tablespoon olive oil
1 medium yellow onion, peeled and chopped
1 large stalk celery, trimmed and diced
4 medium carrots, peeled and diced
1 (15-ounce) can pumpkin purée
3 tablespoons minced fresh ginger
4 cups vegetable broth
1 tablespoon agave nectar
1 tablespoon apple cider vinegar
2 bay leaves
½ teaspoon ground cinnamon
¼ teaspoon dried oregano
¼ teaspoon dried thyme
⅛ teaspoon dried allspice
½ teaspoon ground black pepper
2 tablespoons unsalted pumpkin seeds

1. Heat oil in a small stockpot over medium heat. Add onion and celery and sauté 3 minutes, until they begin to sweat. Add carrots and cook, stirring, 2 minutes, until they begin to sweat.
2. Add remaining ingredients except pumpkin seeds and stir well to combine. Bring to a boil over high heat, then reduce heat to low, cover, and simmer 25 minutes, stirring occasionally.
3. Remove from heat. Remove bay leaves and discard. Use an immersion blender to purée the soup or carefully transfer soup to a food processor and pulse until smooth. Serve warm and top each bowl with pumpkin seeds.

Pumpkin Facts

Pumpkins are a type of winter squash with a hard outer shell and firm inner flesh. Like all winter squash, pumpkins must be cooked before eating. To prepare a pumpkin, simply cut it in half, remove the seeds, and place halves in a microwave-safe bowl. Add an inch or two of water and microwave on high about 20 minutes until tender. Scoop out cooked pulp and use as desired or freeze for later use. Pumpkin is an excellent source of vitamins A and C and fiber.

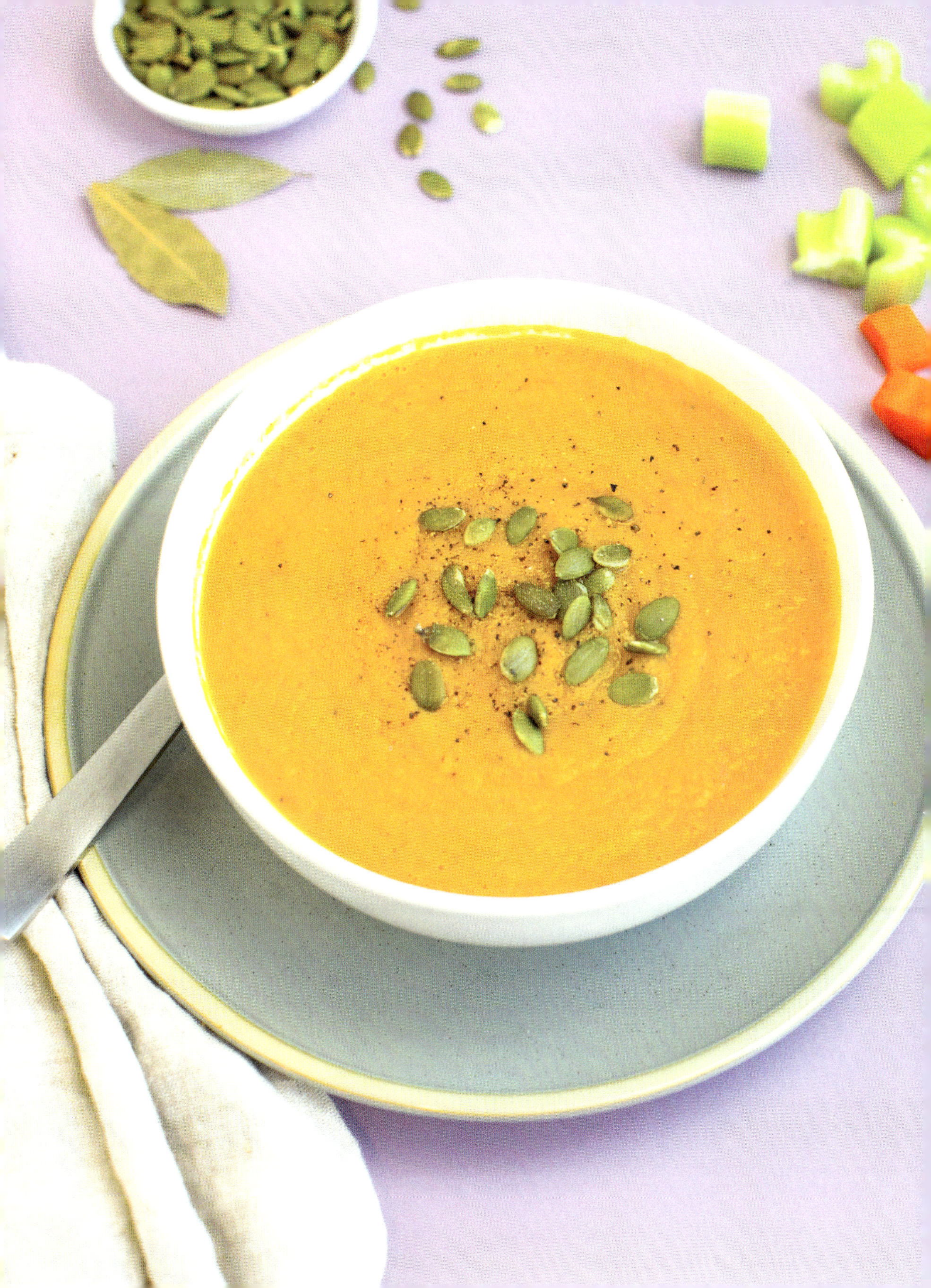

Simple 1-Can Tomato Soup

This soup is so ridiculously easy and delicious, you can make and enjoy it anytime. Partner this recipe with a nice toasted sandwich for a lovely lunch or light dinner.

Serves 4

Per Serving

Calories	112
Fat	4g
Protein	3g
Sodium	860mg
Fiber	3g
Carbohydrates	16g
Sugar	9g

1 tablespoon olive oil

1 medium yellow onion, peeled and chopped

1 tablespoon tomato paste

3 cloves garlic, peeled and minced

2 teaspoons agave nectar

1 (14.5-ounce) can no-salt-added diced tomatoes, with juice

4 cups vegetable broth

3 tablespoons nutritional yeast

1 tablespoon balsamic vinegar

2 teaspoons ground paprika

½ teaspoon dried oregano

½ teaspoon dried thyme

½ teaspoon ground black pepper

1. Heat oil in a large saucepan over medium heat. Add onion and cook, stirring, 5 minutes, until softened. Add tomato paste, garlic, and agave and cook, stirring, 1–2 minutes until paste darkens.
2. Add diced tomatoes, broth, nutritional yeast, vinegar, paprika, oregano, thyme, and pepper and stir to combine. Cover, bring soup to a boil over high heat, then reduce heat to medium-low and simmer covered 15 minutes.
3. Remove from heat and use an immersion blender to purée, or transfer soup to a food processor and pulse until smooth. Serve immediately.

Slow Cooker Minestrone Soup

The ingredients in this soup are fresh and seasonal. Either fresh or frozen green beans work well in this recipe. To stretch the soup further, feel free to add a cup of frozen corn kernels and an extra cup of broth. For the pasta, use small shells or something similar in size.

1 medium yellow onion, peeled and diced
3 medium carrots, peeled and sliced
3 medium stalks celery, trimmed and sliced
3 cloves garlic, peeled and minced
2 cups green beans, cut into 1" pieces
2 (14.5-ounce) cans no-salt-added diced tomatoes, with juice
1 (15-ounce) can chickpeas, drained and rinsed
4 cups vegetable broth
1 bay leaf
2 tablespoons nutritional yeast
2 teaspoons all-purpose seasoning
½ teaspoon dried basil
½ teaspoon dried marjoram
½ teaspoon ground black pepper
⅓ cup small uncooked whole-grain pasta shells

Serves 6

Per Serving

Calories	154
Fat	1g
Protein	7g
Sodium	1,160mg
Fiber	7g
Carbohydrates	30g
Sugar	10g

1. Place all ingredients except pasta in a slow cooker and stir well to combine. Cover and cook on high 5 hours.
2. After 5 hours of cooking time, add pasta, stir to combine, and cover. Cook 45 more minutes, then remove bay leaf and discard. Serve hot.

Cheesy Potato Chowder

This creamy concoction of potatoes, chicken broth, and cheese will make even the staunchest critic a huge fan. White wine adds a lot of flavor, but if you avoid alcohol, substitute an equal amount of broth or a tablespoon or two of rice wine vinegar or white wine vinegar.

Serves 6

Per Serving

Calories	283
Fat	7g
Protein	10g
Sodium	655mg
Fiber	4g
Carbohydrates	44g
Sugar	4g

1 tablespoon olive oil

1 large yellow onion, peeled and diced

3 medium stalks celery, trimmed and diced

2 cloves garlic, peeled and minced

7 medium potatoes, peeled and diced

4 cups chicken broth

⅓ cup dry white wine

½ teaspoon dried thyme

¼ teaspoon ground rosemary

⅛ teaspoon dried basil

½ teaspoon ground black pepper

1 cup shredded Swiss cheese

1. Heat oil in a medium stockpot over medium heat. Add onion, celery, and garlic and sauté 5 minutes, until softened.
2. Add potatoes, broth, wine, thyme, rosemary, basil, and pepper.
3. Bring to a boil over high heat; then reduce heat to low, cover, and simmer 20 minutes, until potatoes are tender.
4. Remove pot from heat. Transfer half of soup to a food processor and pulse until smooth. Return soup to pot and stir well to combine.
5. Add cheese and stir until melted. Serve immediately.

Slow Cooker Split Pea Soup

Unlike dried beans, split peas require no presoaking, so you can assemble this dish any morning and enjoy dinner later in the day. Split peas are high in iron and magnesium, low in fat and sodium, and high in fiber and protein, making this an energy-boosting, metabolism-maintaining bowl of MIND diet goodness.

1 medium yellow onion, peeled and diced
2 medium carrots, peeled and diced
2 medium stalks celery, trimmed and diced
2 medium potatoes, peeled and diced
1 pound (2¼ cups) uncooked green split peas, rinsed
7 cups vegetable broth
1 bay leaf
2 teaspoons all-purpose seasoning
1 teaspoon ground coriander
½ teaspoon ground cumin
½ teaspoon ground black pepper

1. Place all ingredients in a slow cooker and stir to combine. Cover, set to high, and cook, stirring occasionally, 7 hours.
2. Remove bay leaf and discard. Serve hot.

Serves 8

Per Serving

Calories	258
Fat	1g
Protein	15g
Sodium	1,079mg
Fiber	16g
Carbohydrates	50g
Sugar	8g

All-Purpose Seasoning

All-purpose seasoning is a unique blend of herbs, spices, dehydrated vegetables, citrus zest, and sometimes nutritional yeast. Its combination of flavors can replace salt both at the table and in recipes. Benson's Table Tasty is a completely natural, salt-free blend with a salty flavor. It contains no potassium chloride or other chemicals and is sold online.

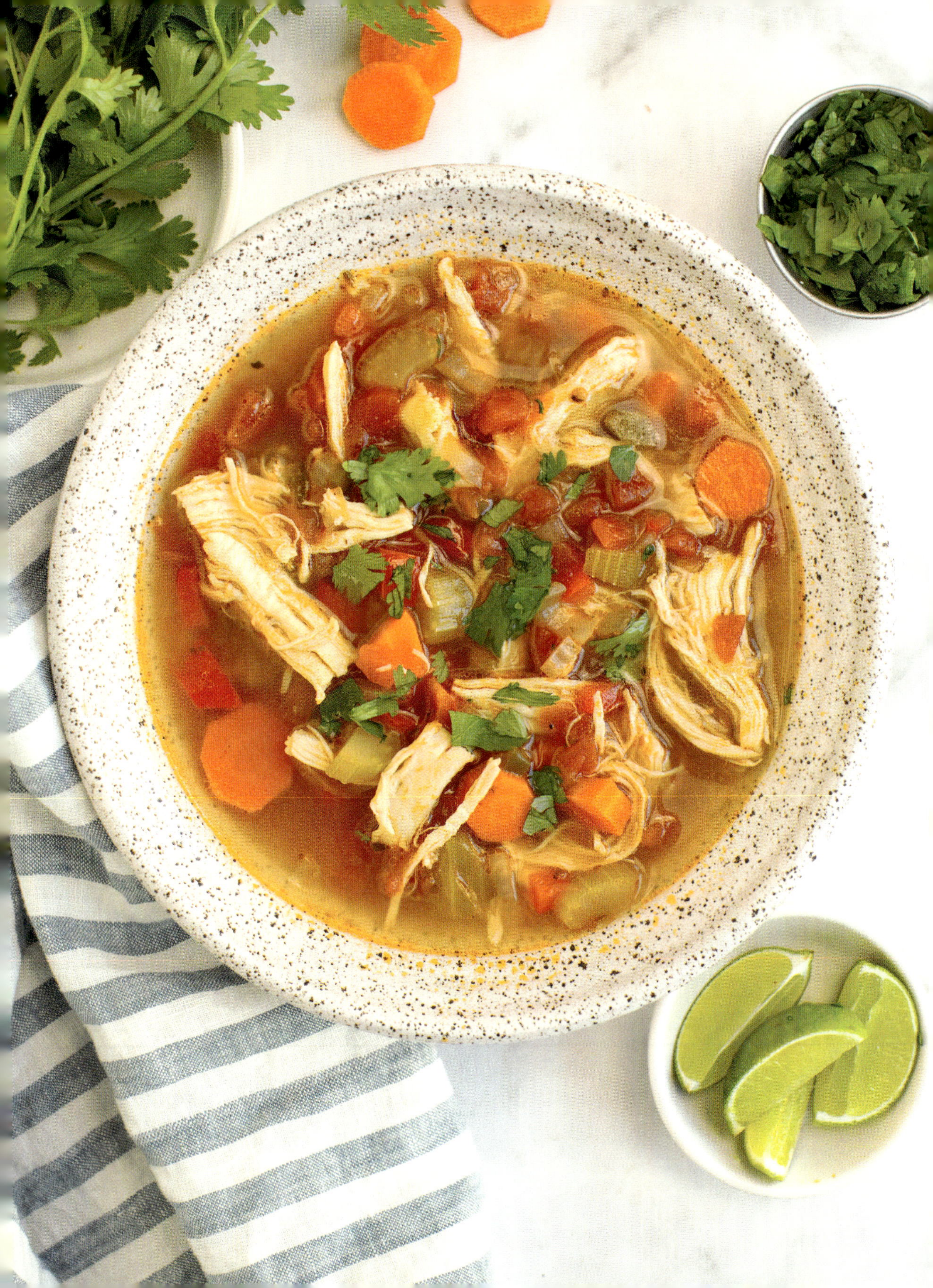

Chicken Soup with Jalapeño and Lime

This soup is brimming with flavor, yet nearly fat-free. For added heft, ladle soup over bowls of cooked brown or wild rice, wide noodles, or quinoa. To reduce the amount of heat, remove the seeds from the jalapeño.

2 cups shredded, cooked chicken breast
1 medium red onion, peeled and diced
3 cloves garlic, peeled and minced
2 medium carrots, peeled and sliced
1 medium stalk celery, trimmed and sliced
1 medium red bell pepper, seeded and diced
1 medium jalapeño pepper, minced
1 (14.5-ounce) can no-salt-added diced tomatoes, with juice
Juice of 2 medium limes
8 cups chicken broth
1 teaspoon ground cumin
½ teaspoon ground coriander
¼ teaspoon dried oregano
½ teaspoon ground black pepper
2 tablespoons chopped fresh cilantro
1 medium lime, cut into 8 wedges

1. In a large stockpot over high heat, place all ingredients except cilantro and lime wedges and bring to a boil.
2. Once boiling, reduce heat to low, cover, and simmer 15 minutes.
3. Remove from heat, ladle into bowls, and garnish with cilantro and lime wedges. Serve immediately.

Serves 8

Per Serving

Calories	109
Fat	2g
Protein	14g
Sodium	977mg
Fiber	2g
Carbohydrates	9g
Sugar	5g

Get the Most from Your Citrus

Before juicing, roll citrus on the counter, pressing down firmly with your hands. The pressure will allow more of the juice to be extracted, and it'll make your hands smell great too! Another tip: When citrus gets old, it often dries out inside. Microwave older fruit for 15 seconds on high to get the most juice from your squeeze.

Chickpea Zucchini Salad

A toothsome combination of flavors and textures makes this salad a favorite in every season, but it's especially tasty in summer made with fresh garden zucchini. If you have fresh dill, substitute 1 teaspoon for the dried. Kelp granules are sold in many supermarkets and health-food stores; they add a distinctive, slightly fishy flavor.

Serves 4

Per Serving

Calories	164
Fat	8g
Protein	6g
Sodium	315mg
Fiber	5g
Carbohydrates	18g
Sugar	4g

What Is Nutritional Yeast?

Nutritional yeast is a type of inactive yeast with a zingy, cheese-like flavor, making it a great substitute for cheese in the MIND diet. The little yellow flakes can be sprinkled on popcorn, pasta, or anything you'd like to perk up. Some nutritional yeast also contains important vitamins such as B_{12}, often found in meat, making it an especially nutritious supplement for vegetarians and vegans.

1 (15-ounce) can chickpeas, drained and rinsed
1 medium zucchini, diced
½ small yellow onion, peeled and minced
2 tablespoons lemon juice
2 tablespoons olive oil
1 tablespoon nutritional yeast
½ teaspoon all-purpose seasoning
¼ teaspoon dried dill
¼ teaspoon herbes de Provence
¼ teaspoon kelp granules

1. Place chickpeas in a medium bowl. Add zucchini and onion and toss gently to combine. Set aside.
2. In a small bowl, add remaining ingredients and whisk together. Pour dressing over salad and toss well to coat. Cover and refrigerate until ready to serve.

Roasted Sweet Potato Salad with Kidney Beans and Peas

This well-rounded salad is pretty, tasty, and healthy! You can substitute walnuts for the pecans if desired and change the salad greens depending on the season: spring mix, arugula, baby spinach, or a blend of herbs and greens. For less spice, reduce the ground cayenne to ¼ teaspoon.

- 2 medium sweet potatoes, peeled and cut into 1" cubes
- 1 small yellow onion, peeled and diced
- 2 teaspoons all-purpose seasoning
- 1 (15-ounce) can kidney beans, drained and rinsed
- ⅔ cup frozen green peas, thawed
- ¼ cup chopped pecans
- 2 tablespoons apple juice
- 2 tablespoons apple cider vinegar
- 2 tablespoons olive oil
- ¼ cup chopped fresh parsley
- 1 teaspoon agave nectar
- 1 teaspoon chili seasoning
- ½ teaspoon ground cayenne
- ¼ teaspoon ground mustard
- ¼ teaspoon ground black pepper
- 6 cups fresh mixed salad greens

Serves 6

Per Serving

Calories	190
Fat	8g
Protein	6g
Sodium	630mg
Fiber	7g
Carbohydrates	24g
Sugar	5g

1. Preheat oven to 425°F. Line a baking sheet with parchment and set aside.
2. In a large bowl, add sweet potatoes, onion, and all-purpose seasoning and toss well. Spread in a single layer on the parchment, place baking sheet on middle rack in oven, and bake 35 minutes until tender. Remove from oven and set aside.
3. In another large bowl, add beans, peas, pecans, and cooked sweet potatoes and toss gently to combine. Set aside.
4. To a small bowl, add apple juice, vinegar, oil, parsley, agave, chili seasoning, cayenne, mustard, and pepper and whisk well to combine. Pour dressing over sweet potato mixture and toss gently to coat.
5. Plate greens and spoon sweet potato mixture over top. Serve warm or cold.

Asian Cucumber Salad

Tangy, crisp, and irresistible, this salad comes together in minutes. Enjoy it immediately or cover and refrigerate; the flavors only improve with time. If you don't have the seedless variety, substitute 2 medium peeled and seeded conventional cucumbers instead. For added appeal, swap in a red onion and sprinkle the salad with toasted sesame seeds before serving.

Serves 4

Per Serving

Calories	107
Fat	7g
Protein	1g
Sodium	388mg
Fiber	2g
Carbohydrates	11g
Sugar	3g

1 large seedless cucumber, sliced diagonally into 1⁄4" slices
1 small yellow onion, peeled, halved, and sliced
1 clove garlic, peeled and minced
2 tablespoons unflavored rice wine vinegar
1 tablespoon olive oil
1 teaspoon sesame oil
1 teaspoon low-sodium soy sauce
1 teaspoon agave nectar
1 teaspoon all-purpose seasoning
1⁄4 teaspoon ground ginger
1⁄8 teaspoon dried red pepper flakes
1⁄4 teaspoon ground black pepper

1. In a medium bowl, add cucumber, onion, and garlic and mix well to combine. Set aside.
2. In a small bowl, put remaining ingredients and whisk well to combine. Pour dressing over salad and toss well to coat.
3. Cover and refrigerate until ready to serve.

Low-Sodium Caesar Salad

This version of the classic salad doesn't require any raw eggs or any anchovies. The dressing is a simple concoction of olive oil, lemon juice, and garlic, whisked with sour cream and Swiss cheese, which is perfect when you decide to have your occasional dairy. This salad is a tangy, creamy, crunchy, and delicious dish that you'll make over and over again.

¼ cup olive oil

2 tablespoons lemon juice

4 cloves garlic, peeled

⅛ teaspoon ground white pepper

½ cup fat-free sour cream

½ cup shredded Swiss cheese

18 ounces (about 9 cups) chopped fresh romaine lettuce

1 tablespoon grated Parmesan cheese

¼ teaspoon ground black pepper

Serves 6

Per Serving

Calories	149
Fat	11g
Protein	4g
Sodium	55mg
Fiber	2g
Carbohydrates	8g
Sugar	1g

1. In a food processor, add oil, lemon juice, garlic, and white pepper. Cover and pulse until smooth. Pour dressing into a small bowl, add sour cream and Swiss cheese, and stir until combined.
2. In a large salad bowl, add romaine. Spoon dressing over top and toss gently to coat. Sprinkle with Parmesan and black pepper. Serve immediately.

Vegetable Pasta Salad with Zesty Italian Dressing

Perfect for potlucks, picnics, and barbecues, this pasta salad will be the hit of the party. The recipe makes enough to serve 12, so halve it if you are feeding a smaller group. You can also make it ahead of time and refrigerate as it will keep well for several days.

Serves 12

Per Serving

Calories	210
Fat	10g
Protein	6g
Sodium	214mg
Fiber	5g
Carbohydrates	25g
Sugar	5g

Salad

- 1 pound uncooked whole-grain rotini (or similar pasta)
- 1 medium red onion, peeled and diced
- 2 cups grape tomatoes, halved
- 1 medium seedless cucumber, diced
- 1 medium red bell pepper, seeded and diced
- 3 cups chopped fresh broccoli
- 1 medium yellow squash, diced
- 1 medium zucchini, diced
- 1 (15-ounce) can chickpeas, drained and rinsed
- ⅓ cup Kalamata olives, sliced

Dressing

- ½ cup olive oil
- ¼ cup apple cider vinegar
- ¼ cup white distilled vinegar
- ¼ cup water
- 3 tablespoons nutritional yeast
- 1½ teaspoons agave nectar
- 1½ teaspoons dried oregano
- 1 teaspoon all-purpose seasoning
- 1 teaspoon dried parsley
- 1 teaspoon garlic powder
- 1 teaspoon onion powder
- ¼ teaspoon dried basil
- ¼ teaspoon ground black pepper
- ⅛ teaspoon dried thyme

1. Make the salad: Cook pasta according to package directions. Drain and set aside.
2. In a large bowl, place onion, tomatoes, cucumber, bell pepper, broccoli, squash, zucchini, chickpeas, and olives. Add pasta and toss to mix. Set aside.
3. Make the dressing: In a small bowl, add all dressing ingredients and whisk well to combine. Pour dressing over salad and toss well to coat.
4. Serve salad immediately or cover and refrigerate until ready to serve.

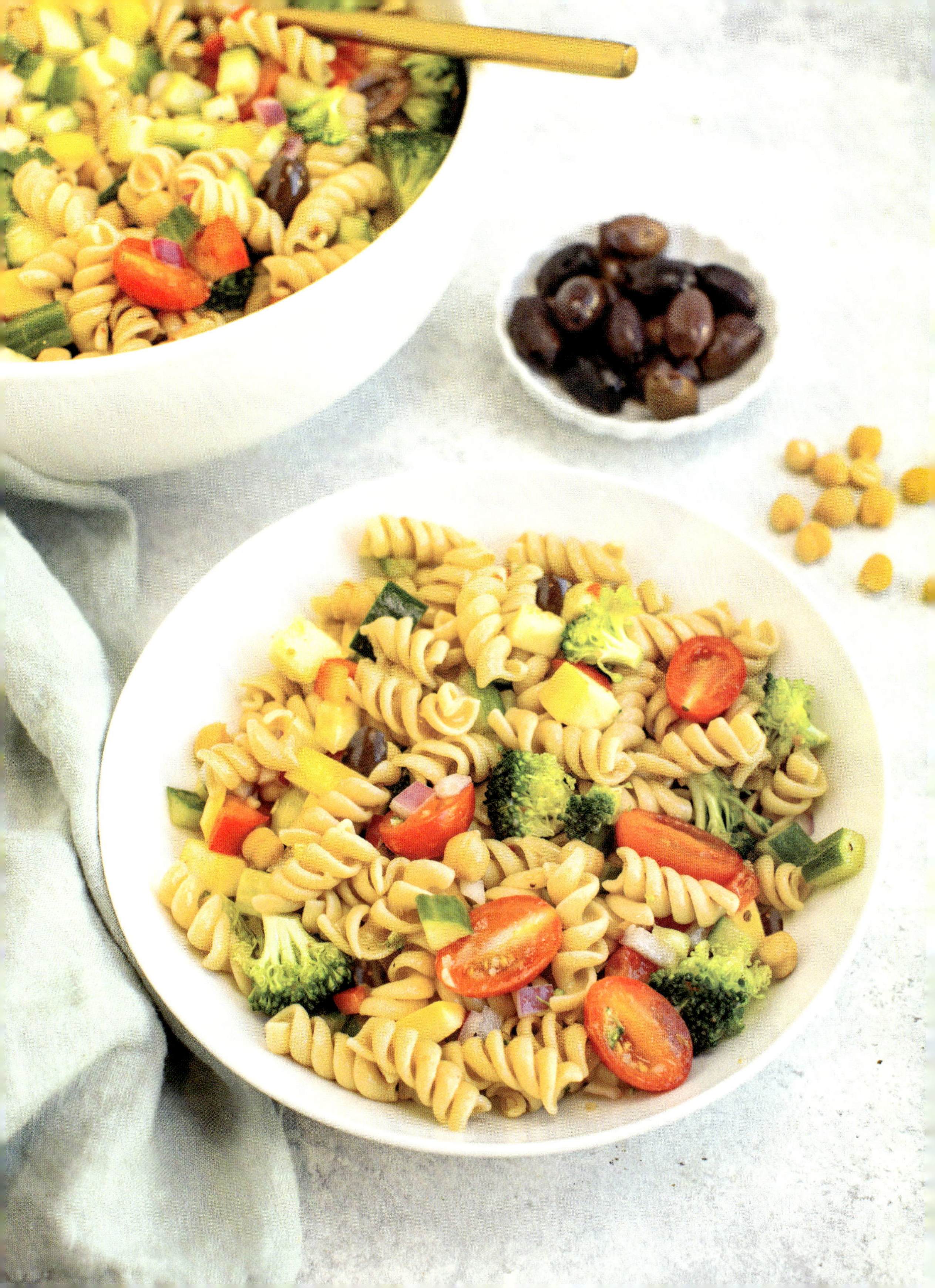

Marinated Mushroom Salad

This salad is delicious as is or you could serve it over greens, partner it with hummus and unsalted chips for a fabulous dip, or use it as a savory topping for pizza. For a spicier version, add ⅛–¼ teaspoon dried red pepper flakes to the dressing.

Serves 8

Per Serving

Calories	89
Fat	7g
Protein	3g
Sodium	97mg
Fiber	1g
Carbohydrates	5g
Sugar	3g

10 ounces fresh mushrooms, diced

1 small zucchini, diced

1 small yellow squash, diced

¼ cup chopped sun-dried tomatoes

¼ cup olive oil

2 tablespoons lemon juice

2 tablespoons apple cider vinegar

2 tablespoons nutritional yeast

1 teaspoon agave nectar

¾ teaspoon garlic powder

½ teaspoon all-purpose seasoning

½ teaspoon dried basil

½ teaspoon ground mustard

¼ teaspoon dried oregano

¼ teaspoon ground black pepper

1. In a large bowl, add mushrooms, zucchini, squash, and tomatoes and stir to combine. Set aside.
2. In a small bowl, add remaining ingredients and whisk well to combine. Pour dressing over vegetables and stir well to coat.
3. Cover and refrigerate at least 4 hours, preferably overnight, stirring occasionally.

Sweet and Tangy Coleslaw with Jalapeño and Lime

This recipe gives run-of-the-mill coleslaw a kick! Celery seed, carrot, and mayonnaise are replaced in favor of minced jalapeño, red bell pepper, and a citrus vinaigrette. It's a tantalizing twist on tradition, as pretty as it is tasty.

¼ cup apple cider vinegar

2 tablespoons lime juice

2 tablespoons olive oil

¼ teaspoon ground black pepper

6 cups shredded fresh cabbage

¼ cup granulated sugar

1 large jalapeño pepper, seeded and minced

1 medium red bell pepper, seeded and diced

2 medium scallions, sliced

1. In a large bowl, add vinegar, lime juice, oil, and black pepper and whisk well to combine. Cover bowl and place in freezer to chill 15–30 minutes.
2. In a large microwave-safe bowl, add cabbage and sugar and toss to combine. Cover and microwave on high 1 minute. Remove, stir briefly, and re-cover. Microwave another 30 seconds or so until cabbage is slightly wilted and has reduced in volume by roughly a third. Carefully drain excess liquid.
3. Remove vinaigrette from freezer and add drained cabbage, along with jalapeño, bell pepper, and scallions. Toss well to combine.
4. Cover and chill at least 15 minutes, then serve.

Serves 6

Per Serving

Calories	112
Fat	5g
Protein	2g
Sodium	15mg
Fiber	4g
Carbohydrates	18g
Sugar	12g

Jalapeño Facts

Used widely in many types of cuisine, the flavor and heat of the jalapeño melds well with many ingredients. To reduce the intensity of the jalapeño, remove its seeds and discard before adding to a dish; the flavor and some heat will remain. Jalapeños are high in fiber as well as vitamins C, B_6, and E.

Salmon Salad with Whole-Wheat Couscous and Dill

This light, fluffy, and flavorful salad can be served warm or cold and even tastes great the next day. You can use up to 2 tablespoons chopped fresh dill instead of the dried.

Serves 4

Per Serving

Calories	359
Fat	10g
Protein	23g
Sodium	1,222mg
Fiber	8g
Carbohydrates	43g
Sugar	6g

Speedy Salmon

When pressed for time, fresh or thawed frozen salmon can be prepared in mere minutes in the microwave. Wash the salmon and pat dry. Place the fillet in a microwave-safe dish and cover the top tightly with plastic wrap. Microwave for 3½ minutes on high. Check the thickest part for doneness; if any bright pink flesh is still showing, cover the dish again and return to the microwave for 30–45 seconds.

1¼ cups vegetable broth

1 cup uncooked whole-wheat couscous

2 tablespoons olive oil, divided

1 medium yellow onion, peeled and chopped

2 cloves garlic, peeled and minced

⅔ cup frozen green peas

1 (7.5-ounce) can salmon, drained

3 tablespoons lemon juice

2 tablespoons nutritional yeast

2 teaspoons all-purpose seasoning

¾ teaspoon dried dill

¼ teaspoon ground black pepper

6 cups fresh mixed salad greens

1. In a 3-quart saucepan over high heat, add broth and bring to a boil. Add couscous, return to a simmer, then cover and remove from heat. Set aside 5 minutes.
2. In a medium sauté pan over medium heat, warm oil. Add onion and garlic and cook, stirring, 3 minutes. Add peas and cook, stirring, another 1–2 minutes. Remove pan from heat.
3. Fluff couscous and add to sauté pan. Flake salmon on top of the couscous. Sprinkle with lemon juice, nutritional yeast, seasoning, dill, and pepper. Toss gently to combine.
4. Serve immediately over greens or cover and refrigerate until serving.

Low-Sodium Greek Salad

This updated Greek salad is perfect for the MIND diet and retains much of the classic taste. Here, a tiny bit of feta enhances the flavor without a huge amount of salt, and the chickpeas add protein and heft. The parsley adds a bright burst of flavor, but if you don't have the fresh herb, feel free to omit.

6 cups chopped fresh romaine lettuce

2 medium cucumbers, peeled, halved, seeded, and roughly chopped

3 medium tomatoes, cut into wedges

1 medium red bell pepper, seeded and diced

1 medium red onion, peeled and thinly sliced

1 (15-ounce) can chickpeas, drained and rinsed

¼ cup sliced Kalamata olives

2 tablespoons feta cheese

¼ cup chopped fresh parsley

2 tablespoons olive oil

2 tablespoons red wine vinegar

2 tablespoons nutritional yeast

1½ teaspoons water

1½ teaspoons lemon juice

½ teaspoon agave nectar

½ teaspoon all-purpose seasoning

½ teaspoon dried oregano

⅛ teaspoon garlic powder

⅛ teaspoon ground black pepper

1. Place romaine in a large salad bowl. Add cucumbers, tomatoes, bell pepper, onion, chickpeas, olives, feta, and parsley.
2. In a small bowl, add remaining ingredients and whisk well to combine. Pour dressing over salad and toss well to coat. Serve immediately.

Serves 4

Per Serving

Calories	265
Fat	12g
Protein	10g
Sodium	516mg
Fiber	9g
Carbohydrates	32g
Sugar	12g

Parsley Facts

Parsley is an easy-growing herb that comes in two varieties, flat-leaf and curly. Use it to add a refreshing taste and color to salads, dressings, and pastas. Parsley contains high levels of vitamins A, C, and K, as well as antioxidants, and may help prevent cardiovascular disease.

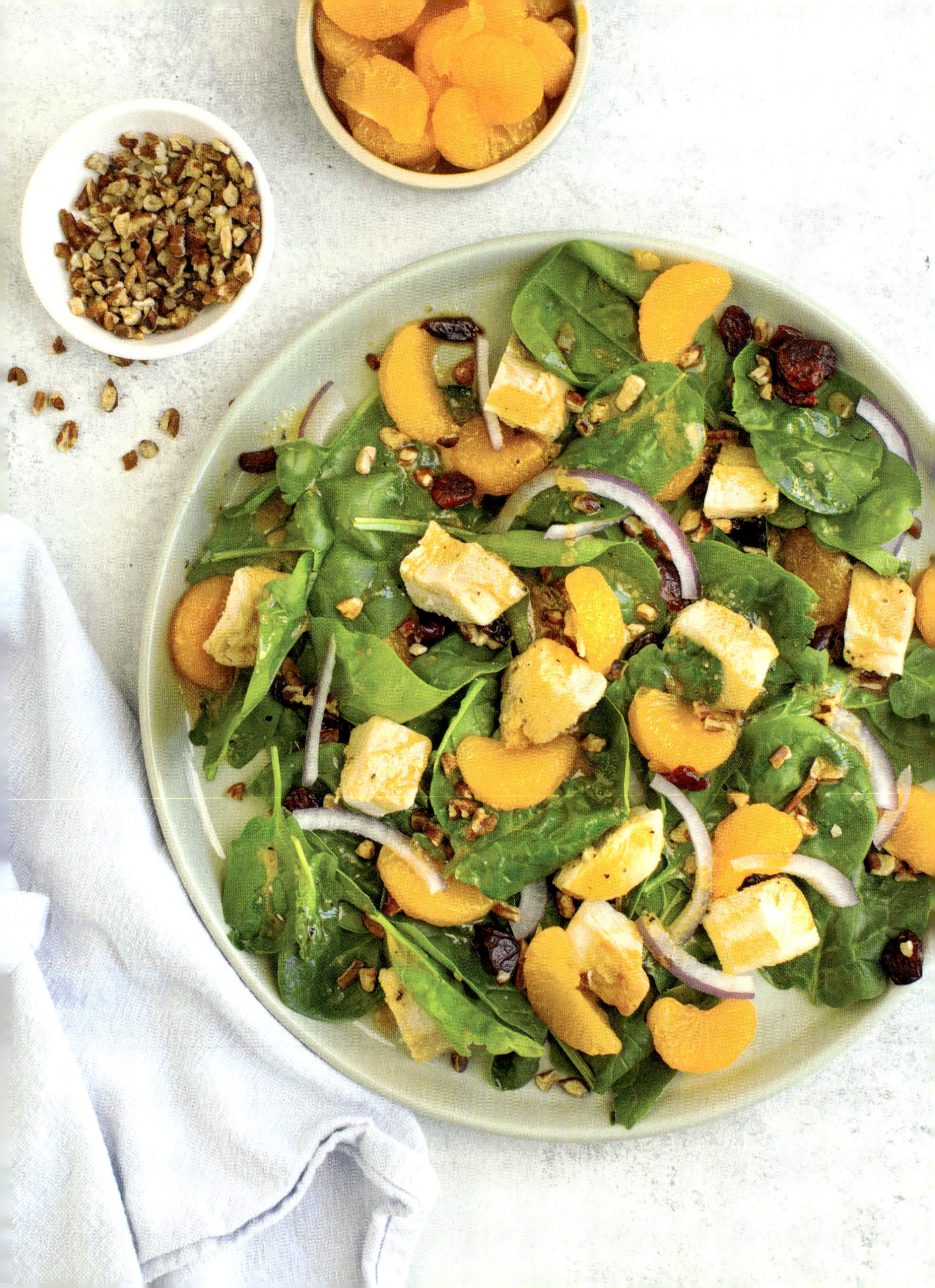

Mandarin Chicken Salad with Spinach and Pecans

This healthy take on a perennial restaurant favorite gives you all the flavor of the traditional dish, but with ingredients that are perfect for the MIND diet. If you don't have red wine vinegar, substitute apple cider vinegar instead.

½ (10-ounce) can mandarin oranges in juice, drained and liquid reserved

2 tablespoons olive oil

2 tablespoons red wine vinegar

1 tablespoon nutritional yeast

1 teaspoon agave nectar

1 teaspoon all-purpose seasoning

1 teaspoon stoneground mustard

⅛ teaspoon garlic powder

⅛ teaspoon ground black pepper

1 small red onion, peeled and finely sliced

¼ cup dried sweetened cranberries

⅓ cup chopped pecans

2 (6-ounce) cooked boneless, skinless chicken breasts, diced

8 cups fresh baby spinach

1. Measure out 2 tablespoons mandarin juice and place in a small bowl. Add oil, vinegar, nutritional yeast, agave, seasoning, mustard, garlic powder, and pepper. Whisk well to combine.
2. In a large salad bowl, place mandarin oranges, onion, cranberries, pecans, chicken, and spinach. Pour dressing over salad and toss well to coat. Serve immediately.

Serves 4

Per Serving

Calories	320
Fat	16g
Protein	30g
Sodium	459mg
Fiber	3g
Carbohydrates	17g
Sugar	11g

Chicken Facts

Chicken's mild flavor and affordability make it a popular protein. When preparing chicken, first remove the skin; this will greatly reduce the amount of fat you're consuming. White meat contains less fat, but dark meat contains a higher concentration of some nutrients. Skinless chicken is an excellent source of protein, vitamin B_6, and minerals such as iron.

Garlicky Kale Salad

The key to this amazing salad lies in preparing the kale. All the handling softens the leaves and allows the flavors to fully permeate the salad.

Serves 6

Per Serving

Calories	54
Fat	3g
Protein	2g
Sodium	84mg
Fiber	1g
Carbohydrates	4g
Sugar	1g

What Is Tahini?

Tahini is a smooth paste made from ground sesame seeds. Its distinctive flavor is used to enhance many Middle Eastern dishes, including hummus, baba ghanoush, and halva. Tahini is sold in the international section of most supermarkets, and once opened it should be refrigerated to prevent spoilage.

1 pound fresh kale, stems removed, leaves chopped (about 8 cups)

3 cloves garlic, peeled and minced

1 tablespoon olive oil

1 tablespoon tahini

1 tablespoon apple cider vinegar

1 tablespoon lemon juice

1 tablespoon low-sodium soy sauce

2 tablespoons nutritional yeast

¼ teaspoon ground black pepper

1. In a large bowl, add kale and massage with your hands for 2–3 minutes to soften.
2. In a small bowl, add remaining ingredients and whisk well to combine. Pour dressing over salad and toss to coat completely, working dressing into salad with tongs 3–5 minutes.
3. Serve immediately or cover and chill before serving. The salad may be made several hours ahead of serving; the longer it chills, the stronger the flavors.

Tuna Salad with White Beans and Tomatoes

Not only is this salad beautiful, it also has an incredible range of flavors. An equal amount of another cooked seafood, such as salmon or shrimp, may be substituted for the canned tuna if desired.

1 (15-ounce) can cannellini beans, drained and rinsed
1 (6-ounce) can tuna in water, drained
1 medium red bell pepper, seeded and diced
1 small red onion, peeled and diced
2 medium stalks celery, trimmed and diced
1 large tomato, diced
2 medium scallions, thinly sliced
1 tablespoon chopped Kalamata olives
2 tablespoons olive oil
2 tablespoons apple cider vinegar
2 tablespoons lemon juice
1 tablespoon tomato sauce
1 tablespoon nutritional yeast
1 teaspoon agave nectar
1 teaspoon all-purpose seasoning
½ teaspoon garlic powder
½ teaspoon dried oregano
½ teaspoon ground mustard
¼ teaspoon ground black pepper

1. In a large salad bowl, add beans, tuna, bell pepper, onion, celery, tomato, scallions, and olives and toss gently.
2. In a small bowl, add remaining ingredients and whisk well to combine. Pour dressing over salad and toss well to coat.
3. Salad tastes best when allowed to marinate, so cover and refrigerate at least 1 hour, then serve.

Serves 4

Per Serving

Calories	210
Fat	8g
Protein	14g
Sodium	844mg
Fiber	9g
Carbohydrates	25g
Sugar	5g

Choose Canned Tuna Wisely

Studies show that many canned tunas exceed the FDA's advisory limits for mercury and should not be eaten often. When buying tuna, opt for chunk light over white albacore, as it is lower in mercury. Some brands contain far lower levels of mercury and higher values of healthy omega-3 fatty acids, so read labels.

Warm Potato Salad with Spinach

This salad shines with a light and flavorful vinaigrette. For added protein, toss in a handful of sunflower seeds or chopped walnuts, or expand the salad into a one-dish meal by adding thinly sliced red onion, fresh green beans, and cooked barley. Fingerlings may be substituted for the new potatoes.

Serves 8

Per Serving

Calories	235
Fat	8g
Protein	4g
Sodium	215mg
Fiber	4g
Carbohydrates	37g
Sugar	3g

What Is Agave Nectar?

Agave nectar is a liquid sweetener derived from the agave plant. It's a clear, light brown liquid, similar in appearance to maple syrup, though slightly thicker. It has a subtle, pleasant flavor and is very sweet, about twice as sweet as cane sugar. Unlike honey, agave nectar is considered a vegan food.

3 pounds small new potatoes
4 cups fresh baby spinach
5 tablespoons red wine vinegar
5 tablespoons olive oil
2 tablespoons water
1 tablespoon yellow mustard
1 tablespoon agave nectar
1 teaspoon garlic powder
1 teaspoon all-purpose seasoning
½ teaspoon dried dill
½ teaspoon dried Italian seasoning
½ teaspoon dried thyme
½ teaspoon ground black pepper

1. Place unpeeled potatoes in a large pot and add enough water to cover by a couple of inches. Bring to a boil over high heat, then reduce heat to medium-high and simmer until tender, about 15 minutes.
2. Remove pot from heat and drain. Cut potatoes into bite-sized chunks. Place potatoes back into the pot and add spinach.
3. In a small bowl, whisk together remaining ingredients. Pour dressing over potatoes and spinach. Toss well to coat and combine. Serve immediately or cover and refrigerate until serving.

CHAPTER 5

Sauces and Dressings

Balsamic Vinaigrette

The combination of balsamic and red wine vinegars lightens the intensity of this classic dressing. The recipe yields ¼ cup, enough for two servings; double or triple the ingredients for a larger or party-sized salad.

Yields ¼ cup

Per Serving (Serving size: 2 tablespoons)

Calories	144
Fat	13g
Protein	0g
Sodium	2mg
Fiber	0g
Carbohydrates	5g
Sugar	4g

2 tablespoons olive oil

1 tablespoon balsamic vinegar

1 tablespoon red wine vinegar

1 clove garlic, peeled and minced

1 teaspoon agave nectar

1 teaspoon ground mustard

¼ teaspoon dried Italian seasoning

⅛ teaspoon ground black pepper

1. Place all ingredients in a small bowl and whisk well to combine.
2. Use immediately or store in an airtight container, refrigerate, and use within 2 days.

Special 6-in-1 Roasting Sauce

This intensely flavorful, spicy-sweet sauce transforms roasted vegetables into irresistible treats. It's delicious on everything from Brussels sprouts and green beans to sweet potatoes and winter squash. It also makes a great brush-on grilling sauce for lean meats and tofu.

Yields 6 tablespoons

Per Recipe

Calories	39
Fat	3g
Protein	0g
Sodium	146mg
Fiber	0g
Carbohydrates	3g
Sugar	3g

1 tablespoon agave nectar

1 tablespoon apple cider vinegar

1 tablespoon lime juice

1 tablespoon low-sodium soy sauce

1 tablespoon olive oil

1 tablespoon sriracha

1. Place all ingredients in a small bowl and whisk well to combine.
2. Use immediately or store in an airtight container, refrigerate, and use within 2 days.

Asian Peanut Sauce

This Asian Peanut Sauce is a creamy, tangy, delicious dressing for salads and bowl meals. This can be tossed with raw or roasted vegetables, whole-grain pasta, quinoa, and more, or used as a dip for grilled meat or tofu. It's so good, you may just want to eat it by the spoon.

3 tablespoons creamy natural peanut butter

2 tablespoons lime juice

1 tablespoon tahini

1 tablespoon apple cider vinegar

2 teaspoons low-sodium soy sauce

2 cloves garlic, peeled and minced

½ teaspoon agave nectar

¼ teaspoon ground ginger

1. Place all ingredients in a small bowl and whisk well to combine.
2. Use immediately or store in an airtight container, refrigerate, and use within 2 days.

Yields ½ cup

Per Serving (Serving size: 1 tablespoon)

Calories	51
Fat	4g
Protein	2g
Sodium	37mg
Fiber	1g
Carbohydrates	3g
Sugar	1g

What Is Vinegar?

Vinegar is produced when an alcoholic liquid is allowed to ferment and the ethanol within it oxidizes. The remaining liquid becomes highly acidic and is what we refer to as vinegar. Balsamic vinegar is made from the pressings (called "must") of white grapes that are first boiled down to form a syrup and then allowed to age. Apple cider vinegar is made from a similar process using apple must.

Lemon Dill Sauce

A delicious dressing for vegetables, green salads, and seafood, this bright and creamy sauce has a lively citrus kick. Kelp granules are sold with the herbs and spices in many supermarkets and natural food stores. When available, you can use 1 teaspoon chopped fresh dill instead of the dried.

Yields 5 tablespoons

Per Recipe

Calories	51
Fat	5g
Protein	0g
Sodium	141mg
Fiber	0g
Carbohydrates	1g
Sugar	0g

2 tablespoons lemon juice

2 tablespoons olive oil

1 tablespoon nutritional yeast

½ teaspoon all-purpose seasoning

¼ teaspoon dried dill

¼ teaspoon herbes de Provence

¼ teaspoon kelp granules

1. Place all ingredients in a small bowl and whisk well to combine.
2. Use immediately or store in an airtight container, refrigerate, and use within 2 days.

Orange Cranberry Sauce

Cranberries, orange juice, and fresh clementine come together in this sweet and tart sauce that's great for holiday dining and so much more. This thick relish is superb year-round as a sandwich topping, addition to breakfast, or garnish for roasted meat.

Yields 2 cups

Per Serving (Serving size: 1 tablespoon)

Calories	33
Fat	0g
Protein	0g
Sodium	0mg
Fiber	0g
Carbohydrates	8g
Sugar	7g

1 cup orange juice

1 cup granulated sugar

3 cups fresh whole cranberries, washed and drained

1 clementine, peeled, segmented, and chopped

1. In a small saucepot, add juice and sugar and stir to combine. Bring to a boil over high heat.
2. Add cranberries and clementine, reduce heat to medium, and simmer 10 minutes, until tender. Sauce will thicken significantly as it cools, so if it appears thin, don't be concerned.
3. Remove from heat, cover, and cool. Serve at room temperature.

Cranberry Facts

Cranberries contain antioxidants and high levels of vitamin C and have been reported to inhibit cancer. But what they're best known for is their ability to protect against urinary tract infections. A substance within the cranberry is thought to prevent bacteria from adhering to the bladder wall, thus preventing attack.

Spinach Walnut Pesto

This scrumptious pesto can be used in a myriad of ways. Stir it into cooked pasta, brown rice, quinoa, or another whole grain. Use it as a spread for sandwiches, crackers, or pizza. Or partner it with raw vegetables and hummus for a party tray. For variety, you can substitute fresh arugula for the baby spinach.

Yields 1 cup

Per Serving (Serving size: 2 tablespoons)

Calories	80
Fat	7g
Protein	2g
Sodium	59mg
Fiber	1g
Carbohydrates	2g
Sugar	0g

2 cups (packed) fresh basil leaves

1 cup (packed) fresh baby spinach

¼ cup chopped walnuts

3 cloves garlic, peeled

3 tablespoons nutritional yeast

3 tablespoons olive oil

1 tablespoon lemon juice

1 tablespoon low-sodium soy sauce

¼ teaspoon ground black pepper

1. Place all ingredients in a food processor and pulse until smooth.
2. Use immediately or store in an airtight container, refrigerate, and use within 2 days.

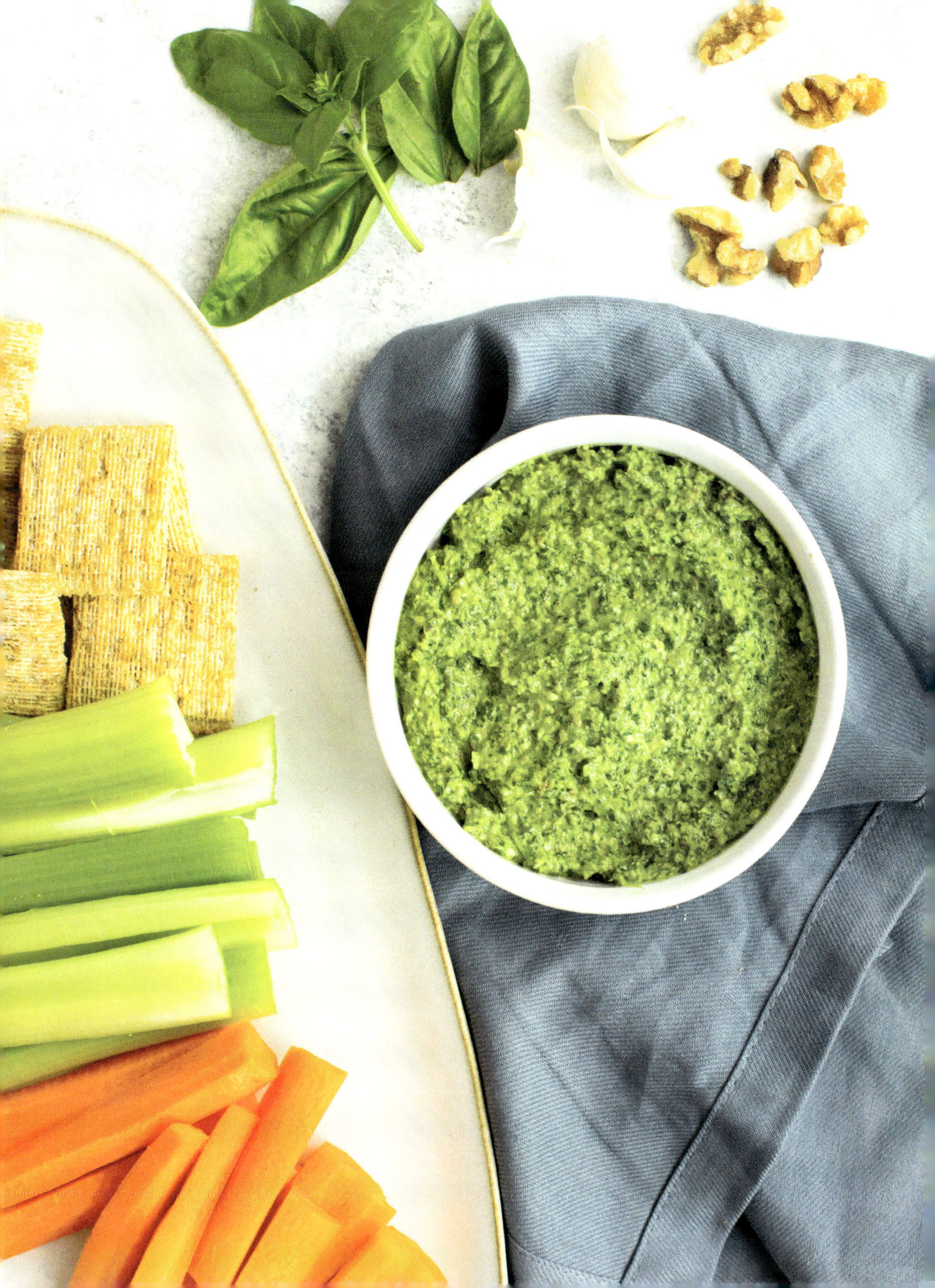

Grapefruit Vinaigrette

This vinaigrette is a light and refreshing dressing with a tangy-sweet taste. Half of a medium-sized grapefruit should yield ¼ cup of juice; use bottled juice if you don't have fresh fruit. Ruby red grapefruit makes a pink dressing as delicious as it is pretty. Drizzle over a mixture of greens, chickpeas, fruit, and sunflower seeds.

Yields ½ cup

Per Serving (Serving size: 2 tablespoons)

Calories	78
Fat	7g
Protein	0g
Sodium	1mg
Fiber	0g
Carbohydrates	5g
Sugar	4g

Grapefruit Facts

Grapefruit is classified by the color of its inner flesh, either white, pink, or red. Grapefruit comes in a range of varieties, some sweet, some much more tartly sour. All varieties contain high levels of vitamin C and antioxidants, as well as lower levels of vitamins A and B_6, and copper. Red and pink grapefruit also contain lycopene, a phytonutrient believed to combat cancer.

¼ cup grapefruit juice
2 tablespoons olive oil
1 tablespoon agave nectar
2 teaspoons red wine vinegar
2 cloves garlic, peeled and minced
½ teaspoon dried marjoram
⅛ teaspoon dried thyme
⅛ teaspoon ground rosemary
⅛ teaspoon ground black pepper

1. Place all ingredients in a small bowl and whisk well to combine.
2. Use immediately or store in an airtight container, refrigerate, and use within 2 days.

Tomato Garlic Dressing

If you're someone who puts ketchup on everything, here's the dressing of your dreams! With its vibrant color and tangy taste, it's great drizzled over salad or served with grilled vegetables, meats, and sandwiches. If you don't have white pepper, substitute ¼ teaspoon ground black pepper instead.

2 tablespoons red wine vinegar

2 tablespoons lemon juice

1 tablespoon tomato paste

1½ teaspoons olive oil

2 cloves garlic, peeled

1 teaspoon agave nectar

⅛ teaspoon ground white pepper

1. Place all ingredients in a food processor and pulse until smooth.
2. Serve immediately or store in an airtight container, refrigerate, and use within 2 days.

Yields about ⅓ cup

Per Serving (Serving size: 2 tablespoons)

Calories	37
Fat	2g
Protein	0g
Sodium	43mg
Fiber	0g
Carbohydrates	4g
Sugar	2g

Homemade Dressings

Store-bought salad dressings offer convenience, but at what cost? Most are filled with fat, excess sodium, and unrecognizable ingredients. Instead of buying commercial dressings, spend money on new and interesting vinegars, oils, and fruit juices. Add garlic, scallions or shallot, fresh or dried herbs, ground or prepared mustard, and some spice, and you've got a world of flavor in mere minutes.

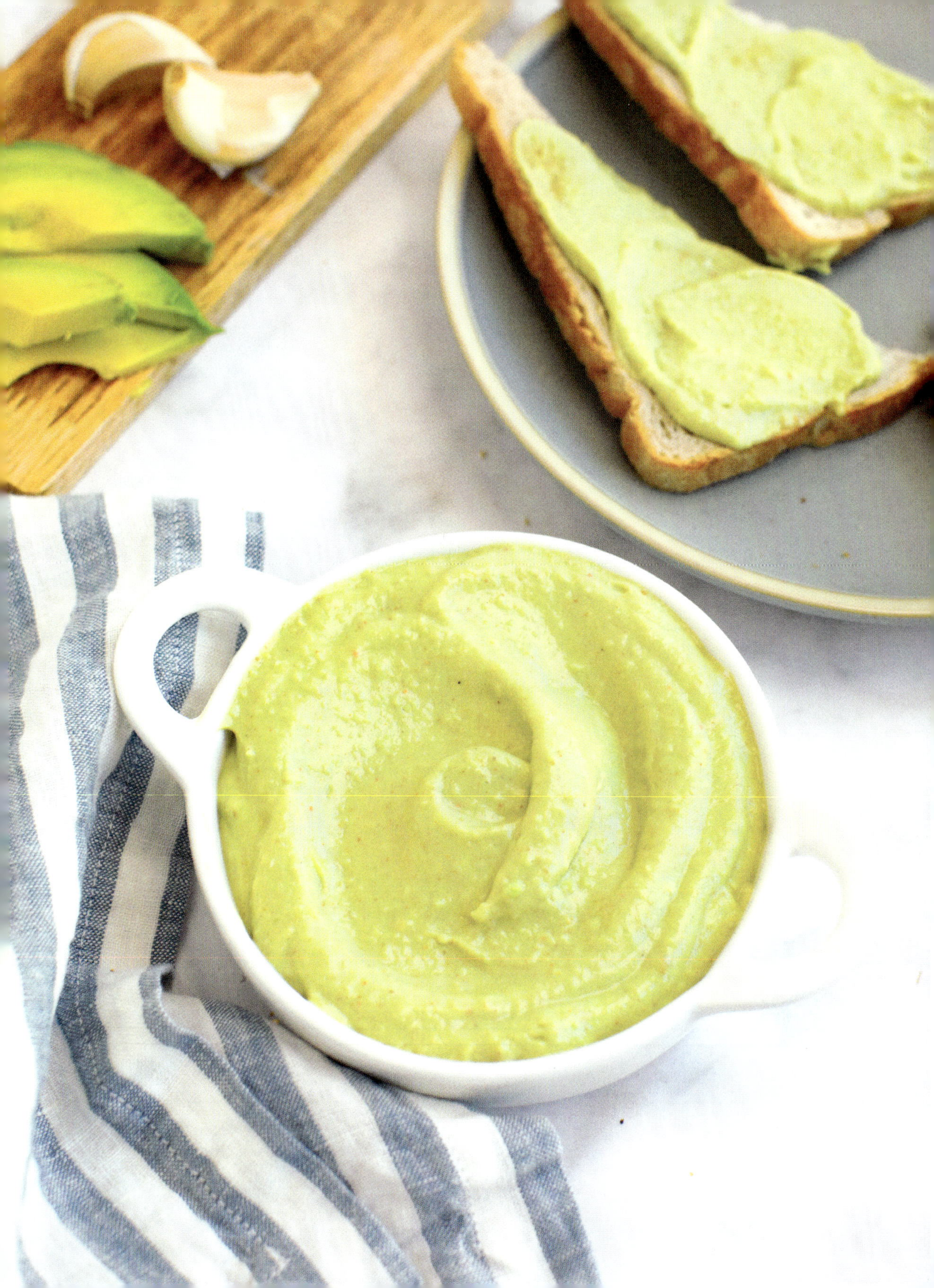

Avocado Whip

This creamy avocado dressing is like a spicy, lime-spiked vegan mayonnaise. It's light, whipped, and fantastically flavorful! Turn any salad into a Southwestern sensation by tossing it with this delicious green dressing. Dollop over nachos or tacos, spread in burritos, or serve with salsa as a dip for tortilla chips. It makes a fabulous sandwich spread and is even great alone on toast.

1 medium ripe avocado, peeled and pitted

4 cloves garlic, peeled and minced

¼ cup tahini

¼ cup lime juice

2 tablespoons apple cider vinegar

2 tablespoons water

1 tablespoon agave nectar

1 teaspoon ground coriander

¼ teaspoon ground cayenne

1. Place all ingredients in a food processor and pulse until smooth.
2. Serve immediately or store in an airtight container, refrigerate, and use within 2 days.

Yields 1⅓ cups

Per Serving (Serving size: 1 tablespoon)

Calories	59
Fat	4g
Protein	1g
Sodium	5mg
Fiber	1g
Carbohydrates	4g
Sugar	1g

Homemade Mayonnaise

This light and creamy mayonnaise uses a liquid egg substitute, eliminating the risk of salmonella. Make this recipe ahead when you have time; it keeps well for a week if stored in a clean, airtight jar in the refrigerator. Adjust seasonings to suit your own taste.

Yields 1 cup

Per Serving (Serving size: 1 tablespoon)

Calories	82
Fat	9g
Protein	0g
Sodium	7mg
Fiber	0g
Carbohydrates	0g
Sugar	0g

Liquid Egg Substitutes

Sold in cartons alongside eggs, liquid egg substitutes such as Egg Beaters are a great way of enjoying the flavor of whole eggs without the fat and cholesterol. In most recipes, you can use 1⁄4 cup of liquid egg substitute for each egg without a discernible difference in taste or texture. Liquid egg substitutes can be frozen as well, making them both healthy and convenient.

1⁄4 cup liquid egg substitute
2 1⁄2 tablespoons distilled white vinegar
1⁄2 teaspoon ground white pepper
1⁄8 teaspoon garlic powder
1⁄8 teaspoon ground mustard
1⁄16 teaspoon ground cayenne
2⁄3 cup olive oil

1. In a food processor, add egg substitute, vinegar, pepper, garlic powder, mustard, and cayenne and pulse until smooth. Scrape down the sides.
2. With food processor running, add oil in a slow and steady stream until mixture thickens.
3. Store mayonnaise in a clean, lidded jar. Refrigerate and use within a week.

Tomato Pasta Sauce

This chunky vegetable-packed tomato sauce is so flavorful! Delicious, healthy, and so easy to make, you may never buy the jarred stuff again. It freezes well too, so feel free to double the recipe and store in an airtight container in the freezer for up to 2 months; thaw before serving.

- 2 tablespoons olive oil
- 1 medium yellow onion, peeled and chopped
- 1 medium red bell pepper, seeded and chopped
- 2 medium carrots, peeled and chopped
- 2 medium stalks celery, trimmed and chopped
- 6 cloves garlic, peeled and minced
- 8 ounces fresh mushrooms, chopped
- 2 cups (packed) chopped fresh baby spinach
- 1 (14.5-ounce) can no-salt-added diced tomatoes, with juice
- 3 (8-ounce) cans tomato sauce
- ¼ cup tomato paste
- ¼ cup red wine
- 2 tablespoons nutritional yeast
- 1½ tablespoons agave nectar
- 2 teaspoons all-purpose seasoning
- 2 teaspoons dried basil
- 1 teaspoon dried oregano
- 1 teaspoon fennel seeds
- ½ teaspoon dried marjoram
- ½ teaspoon dried thyme
- ¼ teaspoon ground black pepper
- ⅛ teaspoon dried red pepper flakes

Yields 8 cups

Per Serving (Serving size: 1 cup)

Calories	148
Fat	5g
Protein	5g
Sodium	753mg
Fiber	4g
Carbohydrates	24g
Sugar	15g

1. Heat oil in a large sauté pan over medium heat. Add onion and cook, stirring, 2 minutes. Add bell pepper, carrots, celery, garlic, mushrooms, and spinach and cook, stirring, 5 minutes, until spinach has wilted and vegetables are starting to brown.
2. Add remaining ingredients and stir well to combine. Cook until the mixture begins to bubble, then reduce heat to low, cover, and simmer 23 minutes, stirring occasionally, until thick and chunky.
3. Remove from heat. Serve immediately or store in an airtight container, refrigerate, and use within 3 days.

Homemade Honey Mustard

This delicious mustard takes only 5 minutes to prepare and yields a sweet and zingy mustard as good as any gourmet brand.

Yields ¾ cup

Per Serving (Serving size: 1 tablespoon)

Calories	55
Fat	3g
Protein	1g
Sodium	1mg
Fiber	1g
Carbohydrates	7g
Sugar	6g

½ cup ground mustard
½ cup distilled white vinegar
¼ cup honey
1 tablespoon olive oil
¼ teaspoon ground allspice
¼ teaspoon garlic powder
¼ teaspoon ground black pepper

1. Combine all ingredients in a small saucepan. Place over medium-high heat and stir constantly until boiling.
2. Reduce heat to medium-low and simmer until mustard begins to thicken, about 5 minutes, stirring occasionally.
3. Pour into a clean, lidded jar; refrigerate and use within a month. Mustard will thicken significantly in the refrigerator, so if it appears thin initially don't be concerned.

Homemade Ketchup

There's no need to purchase commercial ketchup when it's this easy to make at home. This ketchup contains no artificial additives, no artificial preservatives, and no artificial sweeteners, and it's delicious! Season to taste as desired.

3 (8-ounce) cans tomato sauce
5 tablespoons tomato paste
3 tablespoons distilled white vinegar
5 teaspoons granulated sugar
1⁄4 teaspoon garlic powder
1⁄4 teaspoon onion powder
1⁄8 teaspoon ground mustard
1⁄8 teaspoon ground cinnamon
1⁄8 teaspoon ground cumin

Yields 3 cups

Per Serving (Serving size: 1 tablespoon)

Calories	12
Fat	0g
Protein	0g
Sodium	63mg
Fiber	0g
Carbohydrates	3g
Sugar	2g

1. In a large saucepan, place all ingredients and stir until completely smooth.
2. Place pan over medium heat. As soon as the mixture begins to bubble, reduce heat to low and simmer 10 minutes.
3. Remove from heat and pour ketchup into a clean, lidded jar. Refrigerate and use within a month.

Mango Salsa

Ripe mango, garlic, lime, and cilantro flavor this mouthwateringly tasty salsa. When mangoes are out of season, substitute an equal amount of fresh or canned pineapple chunks. Be creative with the recipe and try it out with other fruits, like fresh strawberries, ripe peaches, and garden-ripe tomatoes.

Yields 2 cups

Per Serving (Serving size: ¼ cup)

Calories	35
Fat	0g
Protein	1g
Sodium	1mg
Fiber	1g
Carbohydrates	9g
Sugar	7g

1 medium mango, peeled, cored, and diced

1 medium red bell pepper, seeded and chopped

2 cloves garlic, peeled and minced

1 medium jalapeño pepper, seeded and minced

Juice of 1 medium lime

¼ cup chopped fresh cilantro

1 tablespoon apple cider vinegar

1 teaspoon agave nectar

1 teaspoon ground cumin

1. Place all ingredients in a medium bowl and stir well to combine.
2. Serve immediately or store in an airtight container, refrigerate, and use within 2 days.

Selecting a Ripe Mango

When selecting fresh mangoes, sniff the stem end of the mango for clues to ripeness. Still in doubt? Let your fingers be your guide. Ripe mangoes will yield to gentle pressure, less ripe will give only a little, and unripe will remain hard. Select fruit with smooth, unblemished skin. And don't be fooled by the color of the peel; it has nothing to do with ripeness.

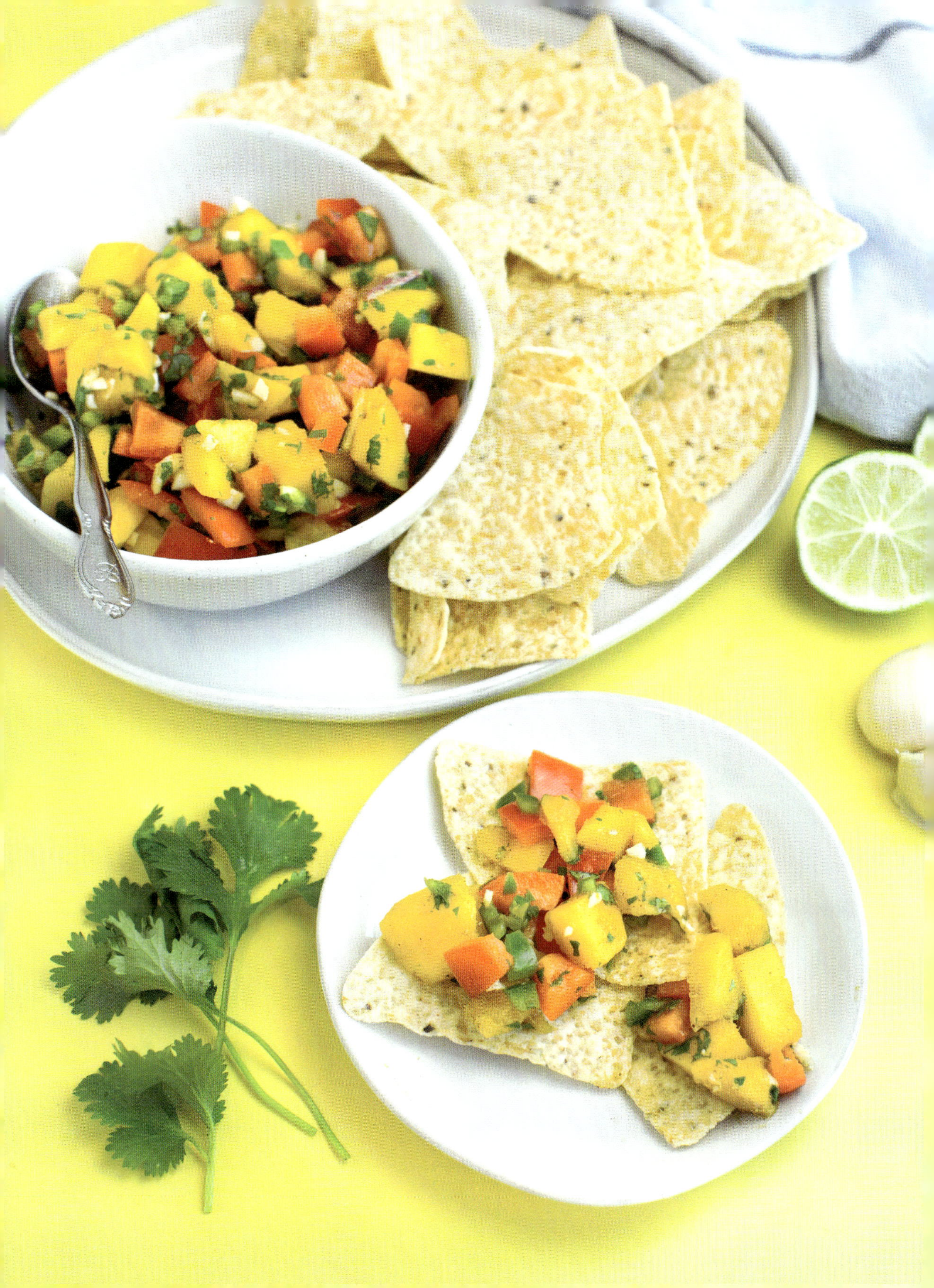

Spicy, Sweet, and Tangy Barbecue Sauce

Fat-free and amazing, this authentic-tasting barbecue sauce is perfect for all of your grilling, basting, and dipping needs. If stored in the refrigerator, this recipe will keep well for a week. For longer-term storage, seal in a freezer-safe container and thaw before use.

Yields 2 cups

Per Serving (Serving size: 1 tablespoon)

Calories	16
Fat	0g
Protein	0g
Sodium	50mg
Fiber	0g
Carbohydrates	4g
Sugar	3g

2 (8-ounce) cans tomato sauce
3 tablespoons apple cider vinegar
2 tablespoons molasses
1 tablespoon honey
1 teaspoon liquid smoke
2 teaspoons onion powder
1½ teaspoons ground cumin
1 teaspoon ground paprika
½ teaspoon garlic powder
½ teaspoon ground black pepper
⅛ teaspoon ground cayenne

1. In a medium saucepan, combine all ingredients and simmer over medium-low heat 10 minutes, stirring occasionally.
2. Remove from heat and pour into a clean, lidded jar. Refrigerate and use within a week.

All-Purpose Seasoning

This recipe tastes great on everything from scrambled eggs to pasta, baked potatoes, popcorn, and so much more. Add additional herbs, spices, or dehydrated vegetables if desired. Feel free to double or triple the recipe and store in a large airtight container for convenience.

3 tablespoons nutritional yeast
1½ tablespoons dried parsley
1 tablespoon onion powder
2½ teaspoons garlic powder
2 teaspoons dried basil
1½ teaspoons dried marjoram
1½ teaspoons ground mustard
1 teaspoon dried dill
1 teaspoon dried oregano
1 teaspoon fennel seeds
1 teaspoon ground paprika
½ teaspoon dried thyme
½ teaspoon ground rosemary
¼ teaspoon ground allspice
¼ teaspoon ground cumin
¼ teaspoon ground sage

1. In a small food processor or spice grinder, place all ingredients and pulse until combined.
2. Store in an airtight container and use within a year.

Yields ½ cup

Per Serving (Serving size: 1 tablespoon)

Calories	15
Fat	0g
Protein	1g
Sodium	4mg
Fiber	1g
Carbohydrates	2g
Sugar	0g

Chili Seasoning

If you have difficulty finding commercial chili seasoning, make your own! After assembling the seasoning, store in a tightly sealed container in a cool, dark place. Although it's convenient to keep spices on the counter, it compromises their flavor.

Yields about ⅓ cup

Per Serving (Serving size: 1 tablespoon)

Calories	19
Fat	1g
Protein	1g
Sodium	6mg
Fiber	2g
Carbohydrates	3g
Sugar	0g

2 tablespoons ground cumin
1 tablespoon ground coriander
2 teaspoons dried oregano
1½ teaspoons ground paprika
½ teaspoon dried red pepper flakes
½ teaspoon garlic powder
½ teaspoon onion powder
¼ teaspoon ground mustard
⅛ teaspoon ground cayenne

1. In a small bowl, place all ingredients and whisk well to combine.
2. Store seasoning in an airtight container and use within 2 years.

CHAPTER 6

Entrees

Lemon Herb–Roasted Chicken

If you crave those aromatic, lemony roasted chickens sold at many supermarkets, then get ready to fall in love. Delicately flavored with fresh citrus and herbs, this roasted chicken will leave you and your dinner companions happy and healthy.

Serves 6

Per Serving

Calories	350
Fat	19g
Protein	34g
Sodium	219mg
Fiber	1g
Carbohydrates	3g
Sugar	1g

1 teaspoon plus 1 tablespoon olive oil, divided

1½ teaspoons dried thyme

½ teaspoon dried basil

½ teaspoon ground black pepper

1 (4-pound) whole chicken

3 cloves garlic, peeled and minced

1 medium lemon, cut into wedges

1 bay leaf

1 small yellow onion, peeled and quartered

½ cup dry white wine

½ teaspoon all-purpose seasoning

1. Preheat oven to 350°F. Lightly oil a small roasting pan with 1 teaspoon oil and set aside.
2. In a small bowl, combine thyme, basil, and pepper. Set aside.
3. Brush the outside of chicken with remaining 1 tablespoon oil, then sprinkle with herb mixture.
4. Place chicken breast-side up in roasting pan. Place garlic, lemon wedges, bay leaf, and onion inside chicken. Pour wine into the pan. Sprinkle outside of chicken with seasoning.
5. Place pan on middle rack in oven and bake roughly 1 hour, until chicken reaches an internal temperature of 165°F and juices run clear when a thigh is pierced with a sharp knife.
6. Remove from oven, let rest 15 minutes, then carve and serve immediately.

One-Pot Chicken and Vegetables

For this dish, chicken breasts are first breaded in a seasoned flour, then browned to a golden crisp, so they retain their shape and yummy coating during cooking rather than simply falling apart like a stew.

1 cup white whole-wheat flour

1½ teaspoons ground black pepper, divided

1 teaspoon garlic powder

1 teaspoon ground paprika

4 (4-ounce) boneless, skinless chicken breasts

3 tablespoons olive oil

1 medium yellow onion, peeled and chopped

3 cloves garlic, peeled and minced

3 medium stalks celery, trimmed and chopped

5 medium carrots, peeled and cut into 1" pieces

6 small potatoes, halved or quartered

1 tablespoon herbes de Provence

½ teaspoon dried rosemary, crushed

1½ cups chicken broth

1. Preheat oven to 375°F. Get out a lidded Dutch oven (or similar oven-safe pot) and set aside.
2. In a medium bowl, add flour, 1 teaspoon pepper, garlic powder, and paprika and whisk well to combine. Dredge chicken breasts in seasoned flour, coating each thoroughly.
3. Heat oil in the Dutch oven over medium heat until it simmers. Add 2 breasts to hot oil and fry just until the outside is golden brown, about 2 minutes per side. Remove from pot, place on towel to drain, and repeat with other 2 breasts. Set aside.
4. To the (now empty) pot, add onion, garlic, and celery. Cook, stirring, 5 minutes, then add carrots and potatoes and stir to combine.
5. Place browned chicken breasts on top, then sprinkle with herbes de Provence, rosemary, and remaining ½ teaspoon pepper. Pour broth over top and cover with lid. Place on middle rack in oven and bake covered 30–45 minutes until carrots and potatoes are soft.
6. Remove from oven and plate each chicken breast with ¼ of the vegetables and ¼ of the broth. Serve immediately.

Serves 4

Per Serving

Calories	490
Fat	13g
Protein	33g
Sodium	486mg
Fiber	9g
Carbohydrates	62g
Sugar	8g

Herbes de Provence

A classic blend of French herbs, typically composed of dried basil, thyme, savory, fennel, and lavender, herbes de Provence gives a distinct flavor to many dishes and is particularly well suited to fowl and seafood. Commercial blends are sold in many supermarkets and online.

Slow Cooker Chicken with Butternut Squash and Kale

This healthy and flavorful one-dish meal is delicious as is, but it's even better served over cooked whole-grain couscous, brown rice, or quinoa. For variety, substitute cubed sweet potatoes for the butternut squash, collard greens or Swiss chard for the kale, and kidney or black beans for the chickpeas. Before serving, sprinkle with chopped almonds or walnuts for added protein and crunch.

Serves 8

Per Serving

Calories	241
Fat	6g
Protein	23g
Sodium	541mg
Fiber	4g
Carbohydrates	22g
Sugar	9g

1 medium butternut squash (about 1½ pounds), halved, seeded, peeled, and cut into 2" cubes

2 pounds boneless, skinless chicken thighs, cut into large pieces

4 cups chopped fresh kale leaves

2 (14.5-ounce) cans no-salt-added diced tomatoes, with juice

1 large yellow onion, peeled and diced

3 cloves garlic, peeled and minced

1 (15-ounce) can chickpeas, drained and rinsed

¼ cup seedless raisins

1 cup chicken broth

1 tablespoon apple cider vinegar

1 tablespoon agave nectar

1 tablespoon ground cumin

2 teaspoons ground coriander

1 teaspoon all-purpose seasoning

½ teaspoon ground cinnamon

½ teaspoon ground ginger

½ teaspoon ground black pepper

1. Add all ingredients to a slow cooker and stir to combine.
2. Cover slow cooker and cook on low 7–8 hours or on high 4–5 hours, stirring occasionally if possible. Serve hot.

Herbed Chicken Paprikash

This flavorful version of the traditional Hungarian dish uses dried herbs instead of salt and substitutes nonfat yogurt for the traditional sour cream. Spinach, mushrooms, and carrots boost the nutritional profile, making this a healthier, more colorful meal that's perfect for those following the MIND diet.

- ½ teaspoon dried oregano
- ¼ teaspoon dried thyme
- ¼ teaspoon dried basil
- ⅛ teaspoon dried rosemary
- 4 (8-ounce) chicken leg quarters, skin removed
- 1 teaspoon olive oil
- ⅓ cup dry white wine
- ⅓ cup chicken broth
- 1 small yellow onion, peeled and sliced thinly
- ⅔ cup sliced fresh button mushrooms
- ¼ cup finely grated carrots
- 4 cups chopped fresh baby spinach
- 2 tablespoons white whole-wheat flour
- 2 tablespoons water
- 2 teaspoons ground paprika
- 2 tablespoons plain nonfat yogurt

1. In a small bowl, add oregano, thyme, basil, and rosemary and stir to combine.
2. Heat a large nonstick skillet over medium heat. Brush both sides of chicken with oil and sprinkle evenly with herb mixture. Add chicken to the skillet and cook on both sides until browned, roughly 2 minutes per side.
3. Add wine and broth to pan and bring to a boil. Reduce heat, cover, and simmer 20 minutes. Add onion, mushrooms, and carrots and cover and simmer 8 minutes. Add spinach and cook 2 minutes more. Remove chicken from pan and place on serving plate. Cover to keep warm.
4. In a small bowl, mix together flour and water and whisk to remove any lumps. Add mixture to the pan and increase heat to medium; bring to a boil and stir constantly. Cook over medium heat and stir until mixture thickens.
5. Stir in paprika. Remove from heat and stir in yogurt. Pour sauce over chicken. Serve immediately.

Serves 4

Per Serving

Calories	330
Fat	12g
Protein	41g
Sodium	266mg
Fiber	2g
Carbohydrates	8g
Sugar	2g

The Beauty of Paprika

Paprika is a powdered seasoning made from ground chili peppers, prized for both its flavor and its beautiful bright red color. Paprika is sold in both hot and sweet varieties. All of the recipes in this book call for the mild (sweet) version.

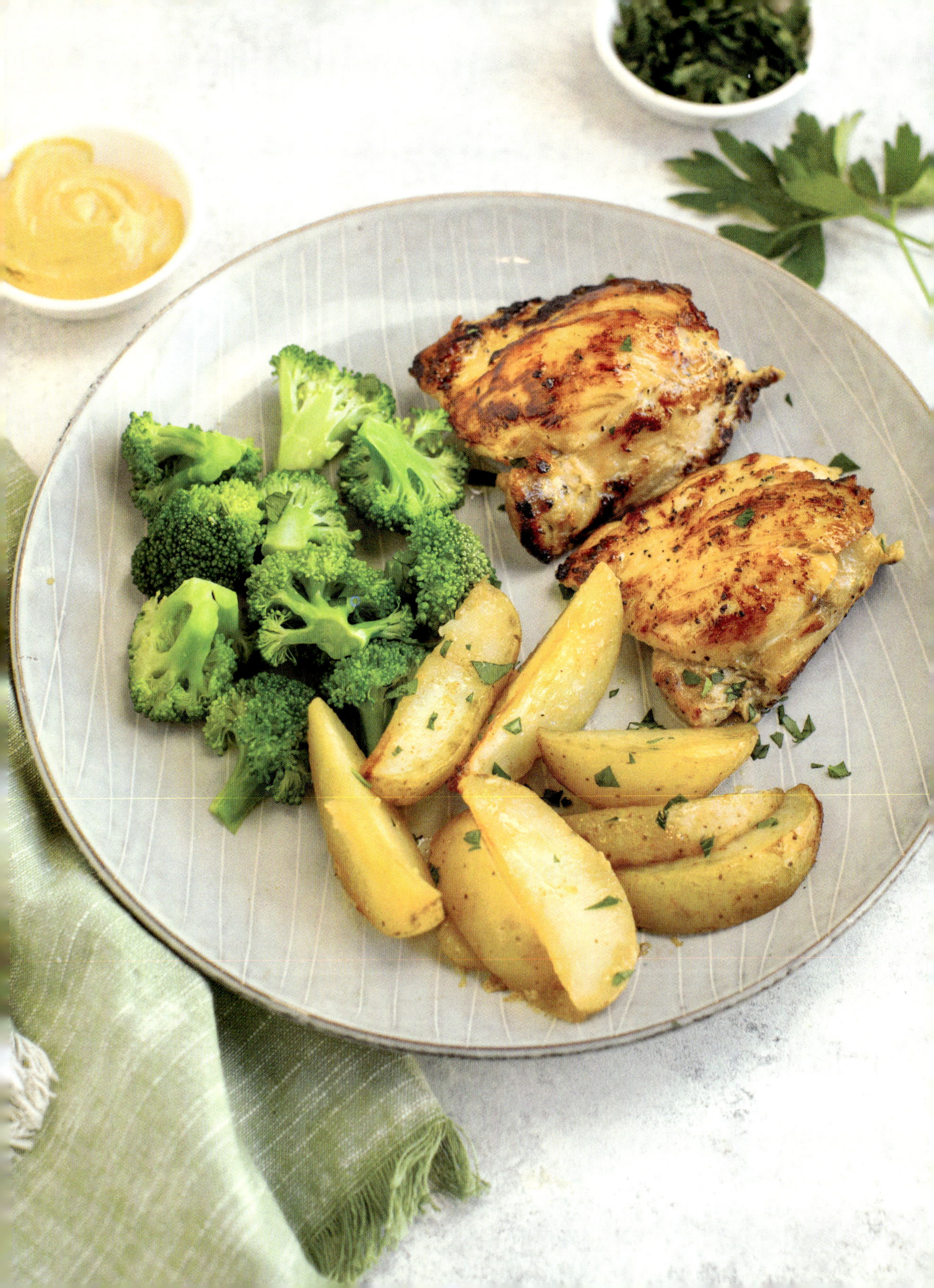

Mustard Maple Chicken with Potato Wedges

The mustard maple marinade, a mix of maple syrup, mustard, olive oil, and apple cider vinegar, is used to marinate as well as to cook the chicken, resulting in a stupendously flavorful meal. Substitute other chicken parts for the thighs if you so desire. Just be sure to cook until the meat is no longer pink when pierced and juices run clear.

1⁄4 cup pure maple syrup

2 tablespoons apple cider vinegar

2 tablespoons olive oil

2 tablespoons yellow mustard

1⁄2 teaspoon ground black pepper

2 pounds boneless, skinless chicken thighs

6 medium Yukon gold potatoes, scrubbed and cut into 8 wedges per potato

1 1⁄2 teaspoons all-purpose seasoning

2 tablespoons minced fresh parsley

1. In a gallon-sized zip-top bag, combine syrup, vinegar, oil, mustard, and pepper. Seal and shake well to combine.
2. Add chicken to marinade bag, seal, and invert several times to coat. Refrigerate 2–3 hours.
3. Preheat oven to 400°F. Oil a 9" × 13" baking dish and set aside. Remove chicken from the refrigerator and set aside.
4. In a large bowl, add potatoes and all-purpose seasoning, and toss well to coat.
5. Arrange potatoes in a single layer in the baking dish. Place dish on middle rack in oven and bake 15 minutes.
6. Remove from oven. Add chicken and marinade to the pan and return to middle rack in oven. Bake 20–30 minutes until potato wedges are tender and chicken has an internal temperature of 165°F and is no longer pink inside. Garnish with parsley and serve immediately.

Serves 6

Per Serving

Calories	373
Fat	9g
Protein	29g
Sodium	605mg
Fiber	4g
Carbohydrates	41g
Sugar	6g

Don't Waste Oven Space

Oven-baked meals are super convenient, and even more so when you simultaneously roast some vegetables. Arrange vegetables in a single layer on a parchment-lined baking sheet and place in the hot oven alongside the main dish. You'll have a delicious, highly nutritious side with little added effort.

Chicken Cacciatore

This classic Italian dish is infused with the flavors of onion, garlic, red wine, and tomatoes. The chicken is first pan-seared to seal in its juices, then slowly simmered in the sauce. Sprinkle with grated Parmesan cheese before serving or pair with pasta and a green salad for an authentic Mediterranean meal.

Serves 4

Per Serving

Calories	271
Fat	9g
Protein	29g
Sodium	530mg
Fiber	3g
Carbohydrates	20g
Sugar	13g

1 tablespoon olive oil

1 large yellow onion, peeled and diced

4 (4-ounce) boneless, skinless chicken breasts

¼ teaspoon ground black pepper

2 tablespoons dry red wine

1 (15-ounce) can tomato sauce

1 teaspoon garlic powder

1 teaspoon dried basil

½ teaspoon dried oregano

¼ teaspoon dried parsley

⅛ teaspoon ground mustard

⅛ teaspoon dried red pepper flakes

1 teaspoon lemon juice

1 teaspoon granulated sugar

¼ cup grated Parmesan cheese

1. Heat a large nonstick skillet over medium heat. Add oil and onion and sauté 5 minutes, until tender. Push onion to the edges of the pan.
2. Add chicken. Sprinkle black pepper over chicken. Pan-fry 2 minutes on each side. Remove chicken from the pan and transfer to a bowl or platter. Set aside.
3. Add wine to the pan. Bring to a boil and cook 2 minutes; use a spoon or spatula to stir well and scrape and deglaze the bottom of the pan.
4. Add tomato sauce, garlic powder, basil, oregano, parsley, mustard, red pepper flakes, lemon juice, and sugar to the pan and stir to combine.
5. Add chicken back to the pan and spoon some of tomato sauce over the top of the chicken. Reduce heat to low, cover, and simmer 45 minutes. Remove pan from heat, top with Parmesan, and serve immediately.

Grilled Jerk Chicken

This dish gives you authentic Jamaican flavor, with MIND diet–approved flavors! Traditional Jamaican jerk seasoning relies heavily on fiery hot Scotch bonnet peppers, while this milder version substitutes ground cayenne instead.

1 teaspoon Jerk Seasoning (see sidebar)

2 teaspoons freshly squeezed lime juice

1 teaspoon low-sodium soy sauce

1 teaspoon olive oil

1 medium jalapeño, seeded and chopped

2 medium scallions, white and green parts chopped

1 teaspoon agave nectar

¼ teaspoon ground mustard

4 (4-ounce) boneless, skinless chicken breasts

1. Preheat an indoor grill or heat a large grill pan over medium-high heat.
2. To a food processor, add jerk seasoning, lime juice, soy sauce, oil, jalapeño, scallions, agave, and mustard and purée until smooth
3. Rub both sides of chicken with spice mixture. Grill 3–5 minutes per side until chicken is cooked through and the juices run clear. Rest chicken 5 minutes, then serve.

Serves 4

Per Serving

Calories	260
Fat	6g
Protein	49g
Sodium	155mg
Fiber	0g
Carbohydrates	3g
Sugar	2g

Jerk Seasoning

To make your own jerk seasoning, combine: 1 tablespoon brown mustard seeds, 1 tablespoon onion powder, 2 teaspoons ground ginger, 2 teaspoons garlic powder, 1 teaspoon ground allspice, 1 teaspoon ground paprika, ½ teaspoon dried thyme, ½ teaspoon fennel seeds, ½ teaspoon black pepper, ½ teaspoon ground cayenne, and ¼ teaspoon ground cloves. Pulse in a small food processor until combined. Store excess in a sealed container in a cool, dark place; it will keep well for up to 2 years. This recipe yields ⅓ cup of seasoning.

Turkey Meatloaf

In this dish, ground turkey is flavored with a tangy herbed tomato sauce and sautéed vegetables and sealed with a homey ketchup glaze. If you don't have bread crumbs, make your own using the directions in the sidebar, or use an equal amount of rolled quick oats instead.

Serves 6

Per Serving

Calories	337
Fat	13g
Protein	29g
Sodium	823mg
Fiber	3g
Carbohydrates	26g
Sugar	11g

Homemade Bread Crumbs

To make your own bread crumbs, crisp several pieces of bread in the toaster or conventional oven. Tear or crumb the toasted bread into tiny pieces. For a finer crumb, pulse the bread pieces in a food processor. Bread crumb substitutes can also be made from finely chopped unsalted nuts, matzo, and salt-free potato chips.

2 teaspoons olive oil, divided

1 medium yellow onion, peeled and diced

2 medium stalks celery, trimmed and diced

1 medium green bell pepper, seeded and diced

1 medium carrot, peeled and shredded

6 cloves garlic, peeled and minced

1½ pounds lean ground turkey

1 (8-ounce) can tomato sauce

1 large egg

¾ cup whole-grain bread crumbs

1 tablespoon molasses

1 tablespoon apple cider vinegar

2 teaspoons all-purpose seasoning

1 teaspoon dried basil

½ teaspoon dried oregano

½ teaspoon dried thyme

½ teaspoon ground mustard

½ teaspoon ground black pepper

¼ cup ketchup

1. Preheat oven to 350°F. Lightly oil an 8" square baking pan with 1 teaspoon oil and set aside.
2. In a medium nonstick skillet, heat remaining 1 teaspoon oil over medium heat. Add onion and cook, stirring, 2 minutes. Add celery, green pepper, carrot, and garlic and sauté 3 minutes. Remove from heat.
3. In a large bowl, add turkey, sautéed vegetables, tomato sauce, egg, bread crumbs, molasses, vinegar, seasoning, basil, oregano, thyme, mustard, and black pepper. Stir with a wooden spoon or your hands until mixture is thoroughly combined.
4. Transfer meat mixture to the prepared pan and smooth top. Spread ketchup evenly over the surface. Place pan on middle rack in oven and bake 1 hour, until meatloaf is cooked through and no longer pink inside.
5. Remove from oven and serve immediately.

Turkey and Quinoa–Stuffed Peppers

Roasted peppers are stuffed with seasoned ground turkey, quinoa, sautéed vegetables, and beans, making each one a balanced meal. Three cups of cooked brown rice, barley, or a similar whole grain may be substituted for the cooked quinoa. Ground chicken may be used instead of turkey if desired.

- 2 teaspoons olive oil, divided
- 3 medium red bell peppers, halved and seeded
- 1 cup uncooked quinoa, rinsed
- 2 cups chicken broth
- 1 bay leaf
- 1 pound lean ground turkey
- 1 medium yellow onion, peeled and minced
- 1 medium stalk celery, trimmed and minced
- 3 cloves garlic, peeled and minced
- 3 cups chopped fresh baby spinach
- 1 (14.5-ounce) can no-salt-added diced tomatoes, with juice
- 1 (15-ounce) can black beans, drained and rinsed
- 1 tablespoon apple cider vinegar
- 1 tablespoon agave nectar
- 1 tablespoon ground paprika
- 2 teaspoons ground cumin
- 1 teaspoon ground coriander
- 1 teaspoon dried oregano
- 1 teaspoon all-purpose seasoning
- ½ teaspoon dried thyme
- ¼ teaspoon dried red pepper flakes
- ¼ cup chopped walnuts
- 3 tablespoons nutritional yeast
- ½ teaspoon ground black pepper

Serves 6

Per Serving

Calories	351
Fat	12g
Protein	27g
Sodium	850mg
Fiber	10g
Carbohydrates	33g
Sugar	8g

1. Preheat oven to 375°F. Lightly oil a 9" × 13" baking pan with 1 teaspoon oil and set aside.
2. Place bell peppers cut-side up in the baking pan. Place pan on middle rack in oven and bake until tender, 30 minutes.
3. While peppers are cooking, in a medium saucepan, add quinoa, broth, and bay leaf and bring to a boil over high heat. Reduce heat to low, cover, and simmer until most of the liquid is absorbed and quinoa is tender, 15–20 minutes. Remove from heat, remove bay leaf, and fluff with a fork. Set aside.

Continued

Continued

4. In a medium skillet, brown turkey over medium heat, breaking up meat as it cooks. When turkey is almost cooked, add onion, celery, and garlic and cook, stirring, 3 minutes. Add spinach, tomatoes, and beans and cook, stirring, 3 minutes. Add vinegar, agave, paprika, cumin, coriander, oregano, seasoning, thyme, and pepper flakes. Cook another 1–2 minutes. Remove from heat.
5. Stir quinoa into turkey mixture and mix well. Remove peppers from oven. Spoon filling evenly into baked peppers. Set aside.
6. In a food processor, add walnuts, nutritional yeast, and remaining 1 teaspoon oil and pulse into a coarse crumb. Sprinkle mixture over stuffed peppers and top with black pepper.
7. Place baking pan on middle rack in oven and bake 15 minutes, until warmed through and lightly browned on top. Remove from oven and serve immediately.

Lemon Thyme Turkey Meatballs

Each bite of these juicy meatballs is heightened with citrus and the heavenly scent of thyme. Serve over whole-grain noodles.

- 1⁄4 cup plus 1 tablespoon white whole-wheat flour, divided
- 1 medium yellow onion, peeled and cut into chunks
- 3 cloves garlic, peeled
- Grated zest of 1 medium lemon
- 1½ teaspoons dried thyme, divided
- 1 pound lean ground turkey
- 3⁄4 cup bread crumbs
- 3 tablespoons grated Parmesan cheese
- 1⁄4 teaspoon ground black pepper
- 2 teaspoons olive oil
- ½ cup dry white wine
- 1¾ cups chicken broth
- 1½ tablespoons freshly squeezed lemon juice

Serves 6

Per Serving

Calories	251
Fat	9g
Protein	21g
Sodium	468mg
Fiber	2g
Carbohydrates	18g
Sugar	2g

1. Place ¼ cup flour in a shallow bowl and set aside.
2. In a food processor, add onion, garlic, zest, and 1 teaspoon thyme and pulse briefly.
3. Transfer mixture to a large bowl and mix in turkey, bread crumbs, cheese, and pepper. Shape into meatballs (2 tablespoons each). Roll meatballs lightly in flour.
4. Heat oil in a large sauté pan over medium heat. Add meatballs and cook until browned, about 5 minutes. Remove meatballs from the pan and set aside.
5. Add wine to the pan, increase heat to medium-high, and cook while scraping up any browned bits, 1 minute.
6. Add broth and bring to a boil. Reduce heat to low and return meatballs to the pan with remaining ½ teaspoon thyme. Cover and cook about 10 minutes, until meatballs are cooked through and no longer pink inside.
7. Remove meatballs again and set aside. Bring sauce to a boil over medium-high heat and cook until reduced to about 1 cup, roughly 5 minutes.
8. In a small bowl, add lemon juice and remaining 1 tablespoon flour and whisk until smooth. Add flour mixture to sauce and simmer 1–2 minutes, whisking constantly until slightly thickened. Remove from heat, add meatballs, and swirl to coat. Serve immediately.

Scallops Fra Diavolo

These rich and meaty scallops are simply sublime. Serve over cooked brown rice, quinoa, or whole-grain pasta for a hearty, healthy meal. Fresh or frozen (thawed) scallops work well in this recipe.

Serves 4

Per Serving

Calories	222
Fat	7g
Protein	16g
Sodium	850mg
Fiber	4g
Carbohydrates	22g
Sugar	12g

2 tablespoons olive oil

1 large yellow onion, peeled and chopped

1 medium green bell pepper, seeded and chopped

4 cloves garlic, peeled and minced

¼ cup red wine

1 (28-ounce) can stewed tomatoes

1 teaspoon agave nectar

¼ teaspoon dried red pepper flakes

1 pound sea scallops

1. Heat oil in a large skillet or sauté pan over medium heat. Add onion and bell pepper and cook, stirring occasionally, 5 minutes. Add garlic and cook 1 minute. Add wine and cook 1 minute.
2. Stir in tomatoes, agave, and pepper flakes and bring to a boil. Reduce heat to medium-low and simmer uncovered 15 minutes until sauce begins to thicken. Stir occasionally. If sauce begins to pop and splatter, lower heat further.
3. Add scallops and cook 5–10 minutes until opaque.
4. Remove from heat and serve immediately.

Baked Tuna Cakes

A moist and healthy twist on traditional crab cakes, these Baked Tuna Cakes are accented with vegetables and a crisp oven-fried crust.

Olive oil cooking spray

2 (5-ounce) cans tuna in water, drained

1 small carrot, peeled and shredded

1 small stalk celery, trimmed and finely diced

1 medium shallot, peeled and minced

2 cloves garlic, peeled and minced

1 large egg white

¼ cup bread crumbs

2 tablespoons mayonnaise

½ teaspoon dried dill

½ teaspoon dried thyme

¼ teaspoon ground rosemary

⅛ teaspoon ground black pepper

1. Preheat oven to 400°F. Spray a baking sheet lightly with olive oil cooking spray and set aside.
2. In a medium bowl, add all ingredients and stir well to combine.
3. Shape mixture into 4 equal patties and place on the prepared baking sheet.
4. Place baking sheet on middle rack in oven and bake 10 minutes. Remove from oven, gently flip cakes, and bake 5 minutes more. Remove from oven and serve immediately.

Serves 4

Per Serving

Calories	138
Fat	6g
Protein	13g
Sodium	264mg
Fiber	1g
Carbohydrates	8g
Sugar	2g

Salmon with Mango and Chickpea Salad

The vibrant colors and flavors of this delicious entree are a treat for the senses. The salmon is baked, leaving it delectably crisp on the outside and juicy within, and it is served with a zesty, sweet, and savory salad. If you don't have any fresh mango, you can substitute another fruit, like pineapple, instead.

Serves 4

Per Serving

Calories	490
Fat	21g
Protein	29g
Sodium	187mg
Fiber	7g
Carbohydrates	45g
Sugar	29g

Chickpeas or Garbanzo Beans?

Chickpeas and garbanzo beans aren't two different things; they're one and the same! The English word "chickpea" comes from the French word *pois chiche. Garbanzo* is the name in Spanish. Chickpeas have a buttery, nutlike flavor that pairs wonderfully with many foods, both sweet and savory. They are high in protein and fiber, very low in fat, and are a rich source of many important vitamins and minerals.

2 medium mangoes, peeled, cored, and diced
1 small red onion, peeled and diced
2 cloves garlic, peeled and minced
1 (15-ounce) can chickpeas, drained and rinsed
3 tablespoons chopped fresh cilantro
Juice of 1 medium lime
4 tablespoons olive oil, divided
1 tablespoon agave nectar
½ teaspoon ground black pepper, divided
1 pound fresh salmon, cut into 4 (4-ounce) portions
1 tablespoon lemon juice
½ teaspoon dried dill

1. In a medium bowl, add mango, onion, garlic, chickpeas, and cilantro and toss to combine.
2. In a small bowl, add lime juice, 2 tablespoons oil, agave, and ¼ teaspoon pepper and whisk well. Pour dressing over mango salad and toss to coat. Cover and refrigerate 1 hour to allow the flavors to mingle and develop.
3. Preheat oven to 425°F.
4. Place salmon in a medium baking dish. Brush with remaining 2 tablespoons oil. Sprinkle with lemon juice, dill, and remaining ¼ teaspoon pepper.
5. Place baking dish on middle rack in oven and bake 12–14 minutes until salmon is opaque.
6. Remove from oven and serve immediately with mango salad.

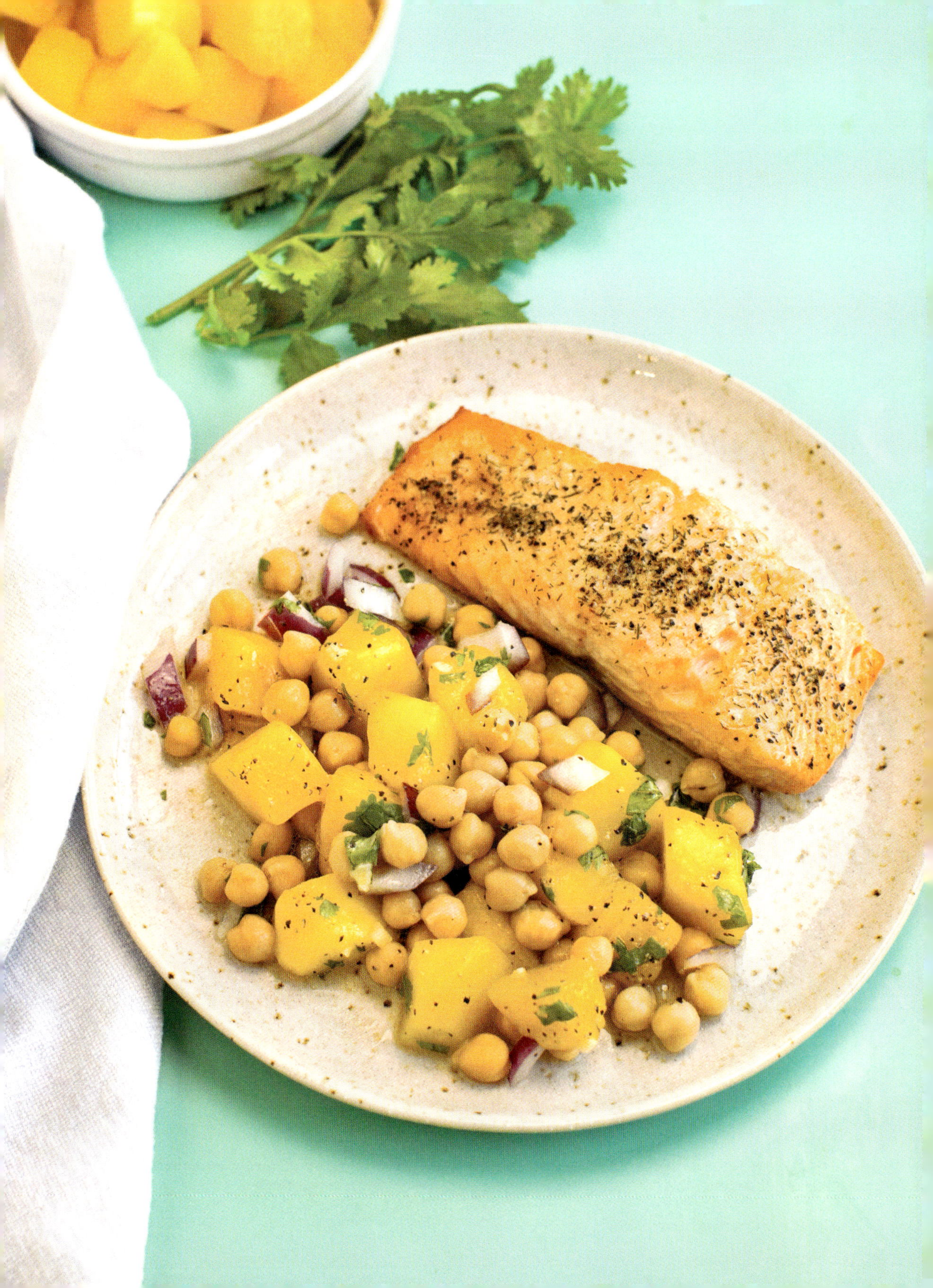

Ahi Tuna with Grape Tomato Salsa

Fish always makes a fresh, light, and easy main course. This recipe calls for broiling the tuna, but it also tastes great grilled. When grilling, 2 minutes per side should be more than enough. Tuna will become tough quickly if overcooked, so be careful.

Serves 4

Per Serving

Calories	176
Fat	4g
Protein	29g
Sodium	55mg
Fiber	1g
Carbohydrates	5g
Sugar	3g

Yellowfin Tuna

Yellowfin tuna, also known as ahi, live in the warm waters of the equator and can grow as large as 400 pounds. Yellowfin tuna is an excellent source of protein, vitamins B_6 and B_{12}, minerals, and omega-3 fatty acids. It is also low in sodium, fat, and calories.

2 cups grape tomatoes, halved
¼ cup finely diced yellow onion
¼ cup finely diced green bell pepper
1 clove garlic, peeled and minced
1 tablespoon apple cider vinegar
1 tablespoon chopped fresh cilantro
½ teaspoon ground cumin
¼ teaspoon ground coriander
½ teaspoon ground black pepper, divided
⅛ teaspoon dried red pepper flakes
1 pound ahi (yellowfin) tuna, cut into 4 steaks
1 tablespoon olive oil, divided

1. Make the salsa: In a medium bowl, add tomatoes, onion, bell pepper, garlic, vinegar, cilantro, cumin, coriander, ¼ teaspoon black pepper, and red pepper flakes and stir well to combine. Set aside. Salsa can be made ahead and refrigerated until time to cook.
2. Preheat broiler. Place tuna steaks on a broiler pan or in a shallow baking dish, brush lightly with ½ tablespoon oil, and sprinkle with ⅛ teaspoon black pepper. Place on top rack in oven and broil 4 minutes.
3. Remove pan from oven, carefully flip steaks, brush with remaining ½ tablespoon oil, sprinkle remaining ⅛ teaspoon black pepper, and return to oven. Broil another 4 minutes.
4. Remove from oven. Plate each steak with ¼ of the tomato salsa. Serve immediately.

Roasted Steelhead Trout with Grapefruit Sauce

The fish is roasted simply, with just a brush of olive oil and dusting of black pepper and then topped with a fruity and bright sauce. The combination of citrus tang, sweetness, and spice is stupendous.

Serves 4

Per Serving

Calories	253
Fat	10g
Protein	25g
Sodium	59mg
Fiber	2g
Carbohydrates	14g
Sugar	12g

1 pound steelhead trout
3 teaspoons olive oil, divided
⅛ teaspoon ground black pepper
2 medium ruby red grapefruits
1 medium shallot, peeled and minced
1 clove garlic, peeled and minced
1 teaspoon minced fresh ginger
2 teaspoons agave nectar
⅛ teaspoon ground cayenne
2 tablespoons thinly sliced fresh basil

1. Preheat oven to 350°F. Place trout in a medium baking dish, brush with 2 teaspoons oil, and season with black pepper. Place dish on middle rack in oven and roast 15 minutes or until internal temperature reaches 145°F.
2. Meanwhile, to prepare the sauce, cut the top and bottom off one grapefruit. Stand it on one end and cut down the sides to remove the white pith and peel. Use a sharp knife to remove each grapefruit segment from its membrane. Cut segments in half and set aside. Juice the other grapefruit and set aside.
3. In a medium saucepan, warm remaining 1 teaspoon oil over medium heat. Add shallot and garlic and sauté 2 minutes.
4. Add ginger, grapefruit juice, agave nectar, and cayenne and stir to combine. Bring to a simmer, then cook until reduced by half, about 10 minutes, stirring occasionally.
5. Remove saucepan from heat. Stir in grapefruit segments and basil.
6. Slice fish into 4 portions, garnish with sauce, and serve immediately.

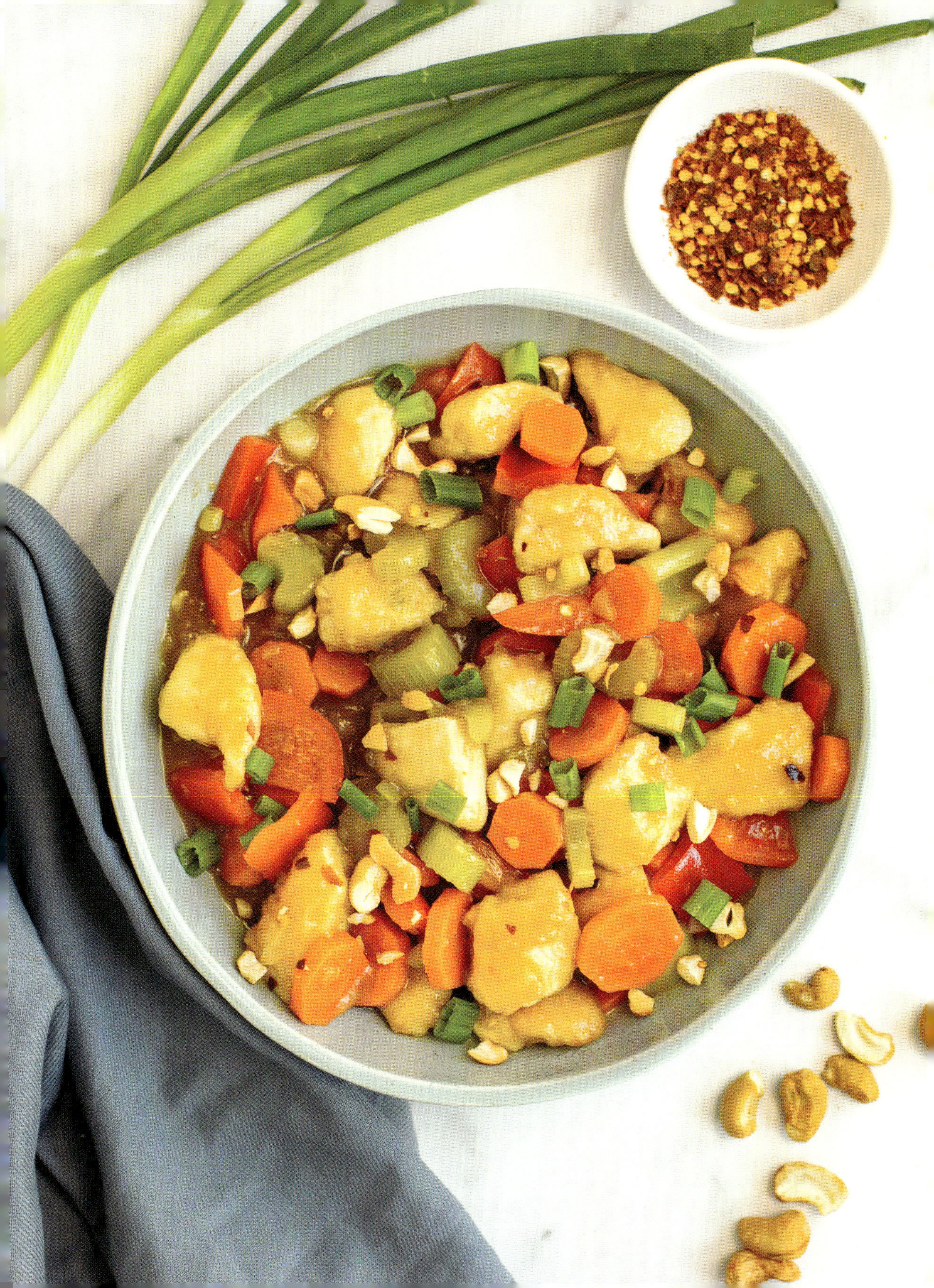

Kung Pao Chicken

The spicy bite of ginger, the tang of rice wine vinegar, the smoky depth of sesame oil, and that certain indescribable something that says "I am Chinese takeout" is all here in this MIND diet–friendly Kung Pao Chicken!

1 cup chicken broth

2 tablespoons low-sodium soy sauce

1 tablespoon balsamic vinegar

5 tablespoons cornstarch, divided

2 teaspoons sesame oil

1 teaspoon granulated sugar

1 pound boneless, skinless chicken breasts, cubed

¼ teaspoon ground black pepper

2 tablespoons olive oil, divided

¼ teaspoon dried red pepper flakes

2 tablespoons minced fresh ginger

6 medium scallions, sliced, whites and greens kept separate

1 medium red bell pepper, seeded and cubed

2 medium stalks celery, trimmed and sliced

2 medium carrots, peeled and sliced

¼ cup unflavored rice wine vinegar

¼ cup unsalted cashews, chopped

Serves 4

Per Serving

Calories	340
Fat	15g
Protein	29g
Sodium	533mg
Fiber	3g
Carbohydrates	23g
Sugar	6g

1. In a small bowl, add broth, soy sauce, balsamic vinegar, 1 tablespoon cornstarch, sesame oil, and sugar. Whisk well to combine and set aside.
2. In a medium bowl, add chicken, remaining 4 tablespoons cornstarch, and black pepper, and toss well to coat using a pair of tongs.
3. In a medium sauté pan over medium heat, heat 1 tablespoon oil. Add chicken and cook until lightly browned on all sides, about 4 minutes total.
4. Add remaining 1 tablespoon oil to pan. Add red pepper flakes, ginger, and scallion whites and cook, stirring, 1 minute.
5. Add bell pepper, celery, and carrots and sauté until they soften slightly, about 2 minutes.
6. Add rice vinegar and scrape bottom of pan to incorporate any browned bits.
7. Give chicken broth mixture a quick whisk, then add to pan.
8. Check chicken; if it is still pink inside, reduce heat and cook a couple minutes more until cooked through. Remove pan from heat, sprinkle chicken with cashews and scallion greens, and serve immediately.

Spicy Tilapia with Pineapple Relish

Tilapia is mild in flavor, meaty, and often inexpensive. For those with an aversion to spicy food, you can omit the red pepper flakes and jalapeño. This recipe is adapted from *Cooking Light*.

Serves 4

Per Serving

Calories	200
Fat	4g
Protein	24g
Sodium	121mg
Fiber	2g
Carbohydrates	18g
Sugar	13g

½ medium fresh pineapple, peeled, cored, and diced

1 small red onion, peeled and diced

1 small tomato, diced

1 medium jalapeño pepper, seeded (if desired) and minced

2 cloves garlic, peeled and minced

2 tablespoons unflavored rice vinegar

2 tablespoons chopped fresh cilantro

2 teaspoons canola oil

1 teaspoon Cajun seasoning

¼ teaspoon dried red pepper flakes

1 pound boneless tilapia fillet

1. Make the relish: In a medium bowl, combine pineapple, onion, tomato, jalapeño, and garlic. Add vinegar and cilantro and stir to combine. Set aside.
2. Heat oil in a large sauté pan over medium-high heat.
3. In a small bowl, combine Cajun seasoning and red pepper flakes and sprinkle evenly over fish. Place fish in pan and cook 2 minutes per side, or until fish flakes easily when tested with a fork.
4. Remove from heat and serve immediately, dividing the fish into 4 portions and plating each with ¼ of the pineapple relish.

Shrimp Creole

This spicy and beautiful shrimp dish is made for special occasions. Serve over cooked brown or white rice.

2 teaspoons canola oil

1 medium yellow onion, peeled and thinly sliced

1 medium red bell pepper, seeded and thinly sliced

2 medium stalks celery, trimmed and thinly sliced

3 cloves garlic, peeled and minced

2 (14.5-ounce) cans no-salt-added diced tomatoes, with juice

1 (8-ounce) can no-salt-added tomato sauce

⅓ cup white wine

½ teaspoon apple cider vinegar

2 bay leaves

2 teaspoons chili seasoning

1 teaspoon ground sweet paprika

½ teaspoon ground black pepper

⅛ teaspoon ground cayenne

1 pound peeled shrimp, tails removed

1. In a medium sauté pan, heat oil over medium heat. Add onion, bell pepper, celery, and garlic and cook, stirring, 5 minutes.
2. Add remaining ingredients except shrimp and stir well to combine. Simmer 10 minutes, stirring frequently. Cover and reduce heat to medium-low if sauce begins to splatter.
3. Stir in shrimp and simmer 5 minutes.
4. Remove from heat and remove bay leaves from pan. Serve immediately.

Serves 6

Per Serving

Calories	146
Fat	2g
Protein	12g
Sodium	565mg
Fiber	4g
Carbohydrates	16g
Sugar	7g

Shrimp Facts

Shrimp come in a variety of sizes and are typically sold by weight and size; for instance, a pound of large shrimp contains roughly 30–35 pieces. Most shrimp consumed in the United States have been processed to some degree and may have added salt. Read package labels carefully and buy fresh, unprocessed shrimp whenever possible.

Seared Sirloin Steaks with Garlicky Greens

If you choose to have red meat occasionally on the MIND diet, then this should be one of the recipes you try. The meat is juicy, perfectly tender, and medium rare; the greens are amazingly delicious, tart, and garlicky with a mustard tang. Serve with roasted potatoes and fresh corn for a truly delectable meal.

Serves 6

Per Serving

Calories	377
Fat	20g
Protein	30g
Sodium	100mg
Fiber	4g
Carbohydrates	13g
Sugar	4g

- 1½ pounds (1"-thick) sirloin steak
- 1½ teaspoons coarsely chopped dried rosemary
- ½ teaspoon ground black pepper, divided
- 4 tablespoons olive oil, divided
- ¾ cup red wine
- 4 cloves garlic, peeled and minced
- 2 tablespoons balsamic vinegar
- 1 teaspoon agave nectar
- ½ teaspoon yellow mustard
- 1½ pounds chopped fresh kale leaves, thick stems removed

1. Preheat oven to 400°F. Take out a rimmed baking sheet and set aside.
2. Trim cut steak into 6 equal portions. Sprinkle steaks with rosemary and ¼ teaspoon pepper.
3. In a large skillet, heat 1 tablespoon oil over medium-high heat. Arrange steaks in the skillet in a single layer (might require two batches) and cook 3–4 minutes per side until nicely browned; only turn steaks once.
4. Remove skillet from heat, transfer steaks to the baking sheet, and roast 4–6 minutes more until medium rare. Remove from oven and set aside to rest.
5. Return skillet to medium-high heat. Carefully add wine, scrape up any browned bits with a wooden spoon, and cook 3–4 minutes until reduced by about half. Add garlic and cook until fragrant, about 10 seconds. Whisk in vinegar, agave, mustard, and remaining ¼ teaspoon pepper. Drizzle in remaining 3 tablespoons oil while whisking constantly.
6. Add kale and cook, tossing, until leaves are wilted enough to fit comfortably in the skillet, about 2 minutes. Cover skillet and cook, tossing once or twice, about 5 minutes until just tender.
7. Transfer steaks to plates and top with greens. Serve immediately.

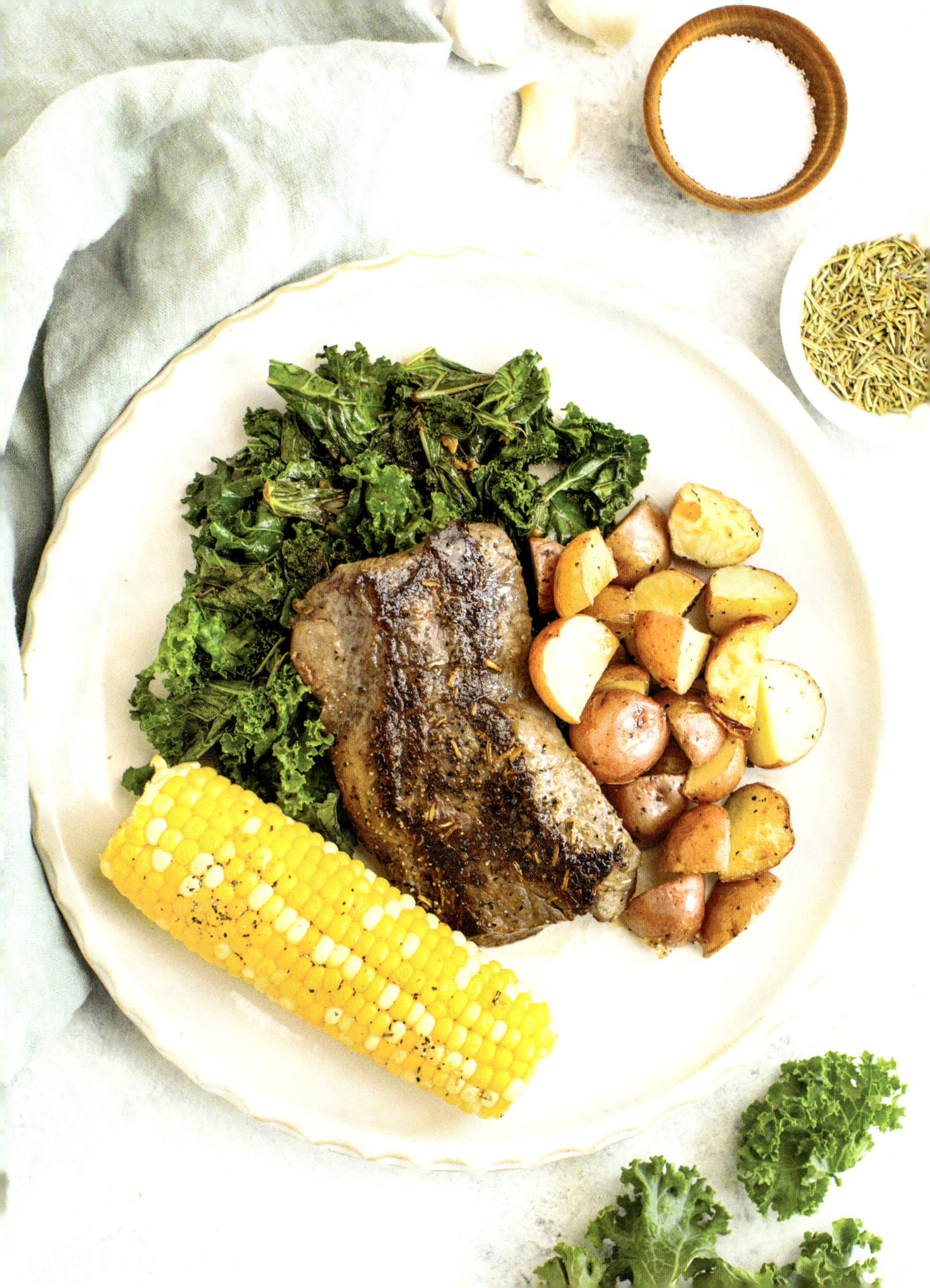

Slow Cooker Pot Roast

The slow cooking renders the vegetables toothsome and the beef tender, which is just what you want when you decide to splurge occasionally and have some red meat. Serve each portion with a generous spoonful of the delicious herb-infused broth and partner this dish with sautéed dark leafy greens.

Serves 8

Per Serving

Calories	399
Fat	11g
Protein	47g
Sodium	720mg
Fiber	2g
Carbohydrates	17g
Sugar	2g

2 cups beef broth

1 cup red wine

3 cloves garlic, peeled and minced

1 teaspoon ground black pepper

1 teaspoon ground mustard

½ teaspoon celery seed

½ teaspoon dried basil

½ teaspoon dried marjoram

½ teaspoon dried oregano

½ teaspoon dried savory

3 medium potatoes, peeled and diced

3 medium carrots, peeled and sliced

1 medium yellow onion, peeled and diced

3½ pounds beef bottom round roast

1. Set slow cooker to low. Pour in broth, wine, garlic, pepper, mustard, celery seed, basil, marjoram, oregano, and savory and stir to combine. Add potatoes, carrots, and onion and stir. Last, place roast into the pot and flip several times to moisten.
2. Place lid on cooker and simmer 8–9 hours, turning roast several times if possible. By the end of cooking time, meat should easily pull apart and vegetables will be fork-tender.
3. Plate beef with vegetables and broth. Serve immediately.

Spaghetti Bolognese

In this recipe, ground beef, sautéed vegetables, tomatoes, herbs, and wine come together in a thick, rich sauce. Substitute your choice of whole-grain pasta for the spaghetti if desired.

1 (12-ounce) package whole-grain spaghetti
2 tablespoons olive oil
1 medium yellow onion, peeled and diced
2 medium stalks celery, trimmed and chopped
2 medium carrots, peeled and chopped
3 cloves garlic, peeled and minced
1½ pounds extra-lean ground beef
1 (14.5-ounce) can no-salt-added diced tomatoes, with juice
2 (8-ounce) cans tomato sauce
⅓ cup red wine
1 tablespoon balsamic vinegar
1 tablespoon agave nectar
1 teaspoon dried basil
½ teaspoon dried marjoram
½ teaspoon dried oregano
½ teaspoon dried thyme
½ teaspoon ground black pepper
½ teaspoon dried red pepper flakes

1. Cook pasta according to package directions. Drain and set aside.
2. In a large skillet or sauté pan, heat oil over medium heat. Add onion and cook, stirring, 2 minutes, until fragrant. Add celery, carrots, and garlic and cook, stirring, 3 minutes until they begin to sweat. Add beef and sauté until browned and cooked through, 5 minutes.
3. Add remaining ingredients and stir well to combine. Cook until mixture begins to bubble, then reduce heat to low, cover, and simmer 25 minutes, stirring occasionally, until thick and bubbly.
4. Remove from heat and spoon over spaghetti. Serve immediately.

Serves 6

Per Serving

Calories	434
Fat	10g
Protein	32g
Sodium	363mg
Fiber	9g
Carbohydrates	57g
Sugar	14g

Cut the Fat

When choosing ground beef or other meats, always buy the leanest cuts possible. When you compare fat for a 4-ounce serving of ground beef, for instance, you can cut your fat intake in half simply by opting for the slightly more expensive 95% lean (5.6g fat) over the 90% lean (11g fat). Leaner meat may be more expensive, but better health is worth the small investment.

Crispy Pork Medallions with Apple Horseradish Sauce

This dish has crispy, panko-coated pork partnered with a stupendous sauce. The flavors of apple and pork meld so fluidly and when you add the bite of sour cream and kick of horseradish, it's out of this world!

Serves 4

Per Serving

Calories	357
Fat	13g
Protein	32g
Sodium	147mg
Fiber	3g
Carbohydrates	27g
Sugar	7g

Pork Facts

Lean pork is considered a healthy meat, especially when consumed in moderation. Pork is an excellent source of protein, vitamins B_6 and B_{12}, and minerals. Its mild flavor is a great partner to most types of fruit, both fresh and dried.

1 cup unsweetened applesauce

¼ cup fat-free sour cream

3 tablespoons horseradish, excess vinegar squeezed out

2 large eggs

1 cup plain panko bread crumbs

½ teaspoon ground sage

½ teaspoon dried thyme

4 (4-ounce, ½"-thick) boneless pork loin medallions

¼ teaspoon ground black pepper

3 tablespoons olive oil

1. In a small bowl, add applesauce, sour cream, and horseradish and stir well to combine. Set aside.
2. Beat eggs in a shallow bowl.
3. In a second shallow bowl, place panko, sage, and thyme, and mix to combine.
4. Lightly season pork with pepper.
5. Dip each loin in egg, then gently press into panko mixture and coat thoroughly.
6. In a large skillet or sauté pan, heat oil over medium heat. Add pork to hot oil and cook until golden and crispy on bottom, 4 minutes. Flip pork and repeat on second side, 3–4 minutes until internal temperature reaches 145°F.
7. Remove pork from pan, garnish with sauce, and serve immediately.

CHAPTER 7

Vegetarian and Vegan

Slow Cooker Thai Red Curry

This one-pot meal is so gorgeous, but it's the taste that's truly fantastic. All-day simmering transforms the vegetables into a softened stew in a light, spicy, citrusy coconut broth. Ladle this curry over cooked brown rice, quinoa, or another whole grain.

Serves 8

Per Serving

Calories	173
Fat	4g
Protein	8g
Sodium	695mg
Fiber	7g
Carbohydrates	28g
Sugar	9g

1 medium yellow onion, peeled and diced

3 cloves garlic, peeled and minced

2 medium carrots, peeled and sliced

1 medium stalk celery, trimmed and sliced

2 cups chopped fresh baby spinach

8 ounces sliced fresh mushrooms

1 cup fresh green beans, cut into 1" pieces

1 medium red bell pepper, seeded and diced

1 medium head broccoli, chopped

1 medium sweet potato, peeled and diced

1 (14.5-ounce) can no-salt-added diced tomatoes, with juice

1 (15-ounce) can chickpeas, drained and rinsed

1 (13.5-ounce) can light coconut milk, shaken well

2 cups water

2 tablespoons Thai red curry paste

2 tablespoons low-sodium soy sauce

2 tablespoons lime juice

1 tablespoon agave nectar

2 teaspoons all-purpose seasoning

1 teaspoon garam masala

1 teaspoon ground coriander

½ teaspoon ground cumin

½ teaspoon ground black pepper

Place all ingredients in a slow cooker and stir well to combine. Cover, set to high, and cook, stirring occasionally, 5–6 hours. Serve hot.

Hearty Vegan Lasagna

This lasagna is every bit as delicious as the classic Italian version. Toothsome mushrooms flavor the tomato sauce, and silken tofu stands in for the ricotta cheese. For an extra-smooth filling, choose a silken variety of tofu; firm or extra-firm will work just fine too.

- 1 teaspoon olive oil
- 2 medium yellow onions, peeled and chopped, divided
- 6 cloves garlic, peeled and minced, divided
- 10 ounces fresh baby bella mushrooms, chopped
- 1 (25-ounce) jar pasta sauce
- 2 teaspoons dried Italian seasoning, divided
- 4 tablespoons nutritional yeast, divided
- 1 teaspoon ground black pepper, divided
- ½ cup vegetable broth
- 8 cups chopped fresh kale leaves
- 1 pound firm tofu, drained
- 1 tablespoon low-sodium soy sauce
- 1 teaspoon all-purpose seasoning
- ⅛ teaspoon dried red pepper flakes
- 1 (9-ounce) package oven-ready egg-free lasagna noodles

1. Preheat oven to 400°F. Take out a 9" × 13" baking pan and set aside.
2. In a large sauté pan, heat oil over medium heat. Add half the onion, half the garlic, and mushrooms. Cook, stirring, until tender, 5 minutes. Stir in pasta sauce, 1 teaspoon Italian seasoning, 1 tablespoon nutritional yeast, and ½ teaspoon black pepper. Set aside.
3. In a large stockpot, heat broth over medium heat. Add remaining onion, remaining garlic, and kale. Stir gently to combine, then cover and cook, stirring frequently, until kale has wilted completely, about 10 minutes.
4. Remove pan from heat and transfer contents to a food processor. Pulse until finely chopped. Add tofu, remaining 1 teaspoon Italian seasoning, 1 tablespoon nutritional yeast, soy sauce, all-purpose seasoning, red pepper flakes, and remaining ½ teaspoon black pepper. Pulse until smooth. Set aside.

Continued

Serves 8

Per Serving

Calories	246
Fat	5g
Protein	13g
Sodium	672mg
Fiber	5g
Carbohydrates	38g
Sugar	8g

What Is Tofu?

Tofu is made from soybeans in a process not unlike the making of cheese. Bean curds are separated from liquid and pressed into blocks. Tofu is sold in two main types. The first, more perishable type must be kept cold. This tofu is submerged in liquid and comes in silken, firm, and extra-firm varieties. Silken-style tofu may also be sealed in shelf-stable packaging so that it does not need to be refrigerated. It comes in varying levels of firmness, from extra soft to extra firm.

Continued

5. To assemble the lasagna, place roughly 1 cup sauce into the pan; spread evenly to coat. Place a layer of noodles over top. Spread ⅓ tofu filling over noodles and smooth evenly. Repeat the process with sauce, noodles, and filling until all are gone. Sprinkle remaining 2 tablespoons nutritional yeast evenly over the top.
6. Cover the pan with a double layer of aluminum foil; carefully pinch the sides to fully seal. Place pan on middle rack in oven and bake 1 hour, until noodles are tender.
7. Remove pan from oven, carefully remove the foil, and serve immediately.

Easy Mushroom and Spinach Quiche

This quiche is the perfect go-to meal for almost any occasion and always gets rave reviews. Fresh baby spinach makes the prep work even easier. Feel free to alter the ingredients to suit your taste, table, or pantry.

½ cup unbleached all-purpose flour

½ cup plus 2 tablespoons white whole-wheat flour, divided

5 tablespoons olive oil

2 tablespoons ice-cold water

1 medium yellow onion, peeled and diced

2 cups sliced fresh mushrooms

4 cups chopped fresh spinach, stems removed

2 large eggs

½ cup low-fat milk

½ cup Homemade Mayonnaise (Chapter 5)

¼ teaspoon ground black pepper

½ cup shredded Swiss cheese

Serves 8

Per Serving

Calories	260
Fat	20g
Protein	7g
Sodium	50mg
Fiber	1g
Carbohydrates	12g
Sugar	1g

1. Preheat oven to 350°F. Take out a 9" pie plate and set aside.
2. In a medium bowl, add all-purpose flour and ½ cup whole-wheat flour and whisk well to combine. In a small bowl, add oil and water, mix well, and pour into flour. Stir until a dough comes together, then gather dough into a ball and place between two pieces of waxed paper. Roll dough out into a large round pie crust, slightly bigger than the pie plate. Carefully transfer the pie crust to the pan; press in and patch as necessary. Set aside.
3. Heat a medium nonstick skillet over medium heat. Add onion and sauté 3 minutes. Add mushrooms and spinach and cook until onion is translucent, spinach is wilted, and mushrooms begin to release their juices, 5–7 minutes. Drain well and set aside.
4. In a large bowl, break eggs and whisk well. Add milk, mayonnaise, remaining 2 tablespoons whole-wheat flour, and pepper. Blend well. Add cheese along with contents of sauté pan and stir to combine.
5. Pour filling into prepared crust. Place pan on middle rack in oven and bake 45–50 minutes until set.
6. Remove from oven, place on a wire rack, and cool slightly, about 15 minutes. Serve warm or cool.

Vegetarian Gumbo

This healthy take on the classic creole dish is filled with brain-boosting vegetables and beans instead of the standard seafood. For more tomato richness, substitute an equal amount of vegetable juice for the broth. Serve over cooked brown rice.

Serves 6

Per Serving

Calories	214
Fat	8g
Protein	7g
Sodium	390mg
Fiber	8g
Carbohydrates	30g
Sugar	9g

What Is Filé Powder?

Filé powder, pronounced /fee-lay/, is a pungent seasoning made from the dried, ground leaves of the sassafras tree. Its unique flavor is added to many Cajun dishes, especially gumbo. In addition to seasoning foods, filé powder also acts as a thickening agent. It's sold at many supermarkets and online.

¼ cup white whole-wheat flour

3 tablespoons olive oil

1 medium yellow onion, peeled and diced

2 medium carrots, peeled and diced

2 medium stalks celery, trimmed and diced

1 medium red bell pepper, seeded and diced

1 small green bell pepper, seeded and diced

4 cloves garlic, peeled and minced

1 (14.5-ounce) can no-salt-added diced tomatoes, with juice

1 cup vegetable broth

2½ cups fresh or frozen (thawed) okra

1 (15-ounce) can kidney beans, drained and rinsed

1 medium zucchini, diced

½ cup tomato sauce

2 bay leaves

1 teaspoon dried thyme

1 teaspoon filé powder

1 teaspoon Cajun seasoning

¼ teaspoon ground cayenne

1. In a large skillet or sauté pan, add flour and oil and whisk well to combine. Cook, stirring constantly, over medium-low heat until brown and fragrant, 10 minutes.
2. Add onion, carrot, celery, bell peppers, and garlic and cook, stirring, 3 minutes. Add tomatoes and broth and stir to combine. Raise heat to medium, cover, and cook 10 minutes.
3. Add remaining ingredients and stir to combine. Bring to a simmer, cover, and cook 15 minutes until vegetables are tender.
4. Remove from heat. Remove bay leaves and serve immediately.

Savory Stuffed Acorn Squash

This tender baked squash is filled with a deliciously seasoned medley of sautéed onion, garlic, mushrooms, and spinach. It's a beautiful meal that looks and tastes impressive but is so easy to make.

Serves 4

Per Serving

Calories	302
Fat	13g
Protein	9g
Sodium	541mg
Fiber	12g
Carbohydrates	43g
Sugar	3g

2 large acorn squash, halved lengthwise, seeds and strings removed

1 tablespoon olive oil

1 medium yellow onion, peeled and chopped

1 medium stalk celery, trimmed and chopped

3 cloves garlic, peeled and minced

1½ cups chopped fresh mushrooms

2 cups chopped fresh baby spinach

¼ cup chopped walnuts

¼ cup bread crumbs

2 tablespoons nutritional yeast

1 tablespoon low-sodium soy sauce

1 teaspoon all-purpose seasoning

1 teaspoon dried basil

¼ teaspoon dried thyme

¼ teaspoon ground black pepper

1. Preheat oven to 350°F. Line a baking sheet with parchment and set aside.
2. Place squash cut-side down on the baking sheet. Place sheet on middle rack in oven and bake until almost tender, 30 minutes. Remove from oven and set aside.
3. In a large sauté pan, heat oil over medium heat. Add onion, celery, garlic, mushrooms, and spinach and cook, stirring, 5 minutes. Add remaining ingredients and stir well to combine. Remove pan from heat.
4. Turn squash halves over on the baking sheet and fill centers evenly with spinach mixture. Place baking sheet on middle rack in oven and bake until hot and tender, 15 minutes.
5. Remove from oven and serve immediately.

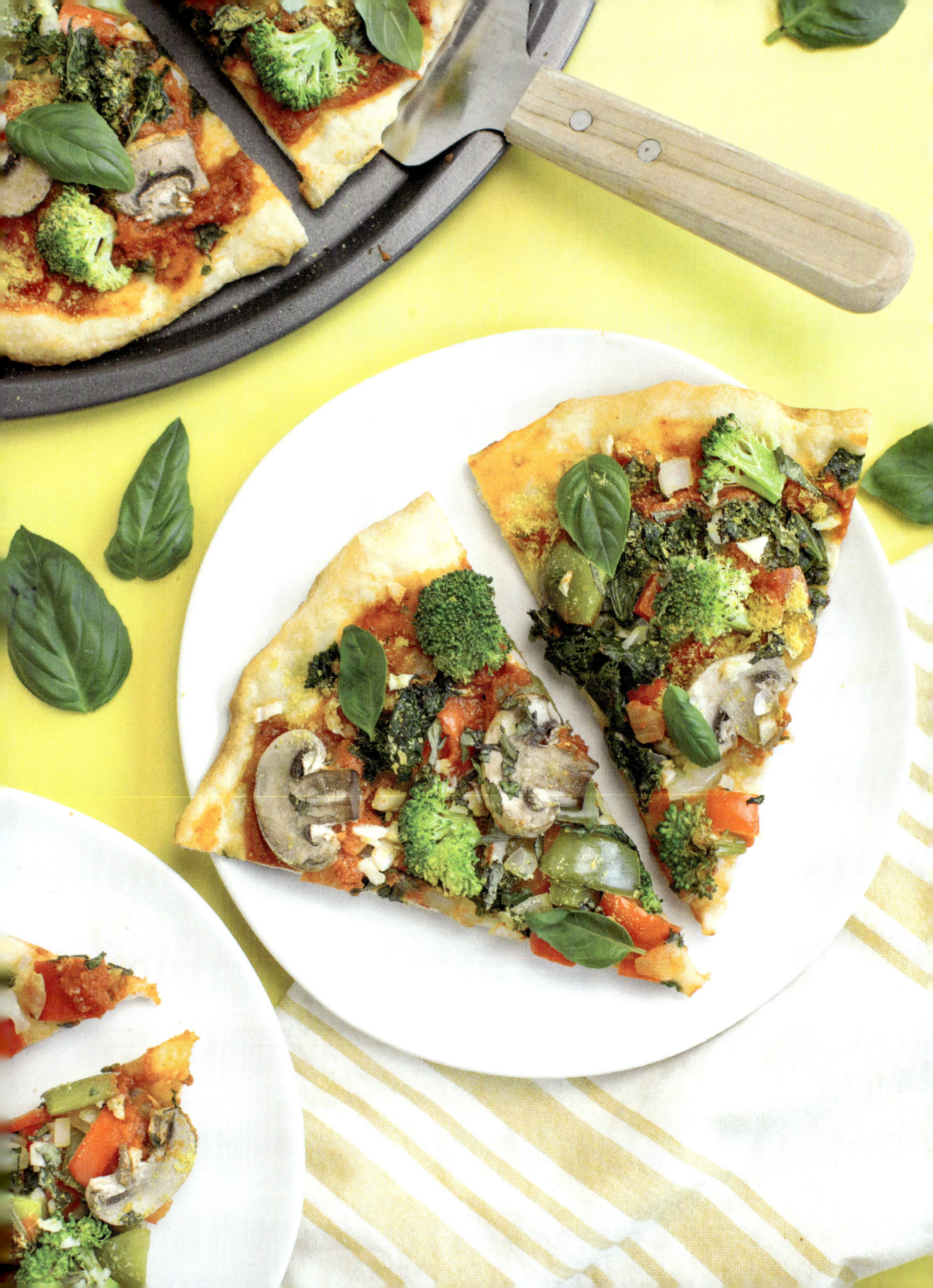

Quick Vegan Pizza

Satisfy your craving for pizza with this beautiful vegan pie. In just half an hour you'll be eating a healthy, satisfying meal that won't compromise your diet. Swap toppings out to suit your own taste; just be sure to weigh the crust down with vegetables during the initial 15-minute baking to prevent it from ballooning up.

- 2 tablespoons ground flaxseed
- 6 tablespoons water
- 1½ teaspoons olive oil
- 1 medium yellow onion, peeled and diced
- 1 medium red bell pepper, seeded and diced
- 1 medium green bell pepper, seeded and diced
- 2 cups chopped fresh kale leaves
- 1 cup white whole-wheat flour
- 1 tablespoon baking powder
- 1 tablespoon beet sugar
- 1 teaspoon all-purpose seasoning
- 1 teaspoon dried Italian seasoning
- ½ teaspoon garlic powder
- ⅔ cup unsweetened almond milk
- ½ cup jarred pasta sauce
- 2 cloves garlic, peeled and minced
- 2 tablespoons chopped fresh basil
- 1 cup chopped fresh broccoli
- ½ cup sliced fresh mushrooms
- 1 tablespoon nutritional yeast
- ½ teaspoon ground black pepper

1. Preheat oven to 450°F. Grease and flour a 12" pizza pan and set aside.
2. In a small bowl, add flaxseed and water and stir to combine. Let rest a few minutes to thicken.
3. In a large sauté pan, heat oil over medium heat. Add onion, bell peppers, and kale and cook, stirring, 5 minutes. Remove from heat and set aside.
4. In a medium bowl, add flour, baking powder, sugar, all-purpose seasoning, Italian seasoning, and garlic powder and whisk well to combine. Add flaxseed mixture and milk and stir just until combined into a batter.

Continued

Serves 4

Per Serving

Calories	224
Fat	5g
Protein	8g
Sodium	900mg
Fiber	8g
Carbohydrates	39g
Sugar	9g

Easy Greasing

The simplest way to grease and flour a pizza pan is by using olive oil cooking spray. Spray pan lightly with oil, add 1 tablespoon flour, then tap pan and tilt to disperse the flour. After the surface is evenly coated, tip pan over the sink, compost bin, or trash can and tap lightly to remove excess flour.

Continued

5. Transfer batter into prepared pizza pan and spread evenly to the edges. The dough may be a bit thick and unwieldy; just spread and smooth away holes as they arise.
6. Spoon sautéed vegetables evenly over the surface of dough. Place pan on middle rack in oven and bake 15 minutes.
7. Remove pan from oven and spread sauce evenly over crust. Top with remaining ingredients, return to oven, and bake another 5 minutes.
8. Remove pan from oven. Cut pizza into 8 slices and serve immediately.

Ratatouille

This version of the classic dish is bursting with the intermingling flavors of fresh summer vegetables. If you have fresh herbs, feel free to use them, just add three times the amount of any fresh herb in place of the dried.

- 2 tablespoons olive oil
- 2 medium yellow onions, peeled and diced
- 6 cloves garlic, peeled and minced
- 1 medium red bell pepper, seeded and diced
- 1 (14.5-ounce) can no-salt-added diced tomatoes, with juice
- 2 (8-ounce) cans tomato sauce
- 2 tablespoons tomato paste
- 1 tablespoon agave nectar
- 1 tablespoon balsamic vinegar
- 1 teaspoon dried basil
- 3⁄4 teaspoon dried marjoram
- 1⁄2 teaspoon dried oregano
- 1⁄2 teaspoon fennel seeds
- 1⁄2 teaspoon ground black pepper
- 1⁄4 teaspoon dried thyme
- 1 large eggplant, peeled and sliced lengthwise into strips
- 2 medium zucchini, sliced into thin rounds
- 2 medium yellow squash, sliced into thin rounds
- 3 tablespoons nutritional yeast

Serves 8

Per Serving

Calories	146
Fat	5g
Protein	5g
Sodium	5mg
Fiber	6g
Carbohydrates	24g
Sugar	15g

1. Preheat oven to 375°F. Take out a 9" × 13" oven-safe casserole dish and set aside.
2. In a large skillet or sauté pan, heat oil over medium heat. Add onion and garlic and sauté 3 minutes. Add bell pepper and diced tomatoes and cook, stirring, 5 minutes. Add tomato sauce, tomato paste, agave, vinegar, basil, marjoram, oregano, fennel, black pepper, and thyme. Reduce heat to medium-low and simmer 10 minutes, stirring frequently. Remove from heat.
3. Assemble ratatouille in layers, like a lasagna. First, spoon some sauce into the bottom of the pan. Arrange eggplant over top, then cover with a thin layer of sauce. Arrange zucchini next and top with another thin layer of sauce. Then arrange squash and top with a thin layer of sauce. Repeat with any remaining vegetables. Top finally with remaining sauce and nutritional yeast.
4. Cover the pan tightly with aluminum foil. Place dish on middle rack in oven and bake 1 hour, until tender and bubbling.
5. Carefully remove pan from oven and place on a wire rack to cool slightly before serving. Serve hot, warm, or at room temperature.

Spicy Noodles

This is a great go-to recipe when time is tight. It's quick, filling, and delicious. For less spice, reduce the red pepper flakes to ¼ teaspoon. This recipe makes a very "dry" noodle; if you prefer a more liquid sauce, add additional broth.

Serves 6

Per Serving

Calories	229
Fat	2g
Protein	10g
Sodium	203mg
Fiber	9g
Carbohydrates	46g
Sugar	4g

1 (12-ounce) package whole-grain spaghetti
2 teaspoons olive oil
1 small yellow onion, peeled and chopped
3 cloves garlic, peeled and minced
1 medium carrot, peeled and chopped
1 medium red bell pepper, seeded and chopped
3 cups chopped fresh broccoli
½ cup vegetable broth
3 tablespoons apple cider vinegar
1½ tablespoons low-sodium soy sauce
1½ teaspoons ground paprika
½ teaspoon ground ginger
½ teaspoon dried red pepper flakes
⅛ teaspoon ground black pepper

1. Cook spaghetti according to package directions.
2. In a large sauté pan or skillet, heat oil over medium heat. Add onion and cook, stirring, 2 minutes, until it begins to sweat. Add garlic, carrot, bell pepper, and broccoli and cook, stirring, 5 minutes, until tender. Remove pan from heat.
3. Drain pasta and add to sauté pan. Add remaining ingredients and toss for a minute to fully coat and combine. Serve immediately.

Oven-Baked Spinach Burgers

These spinach- and onion-flecked burgers, filled with brain-boosting vitamin K, are perfect to eat on the MIND diet. For a vegan version, substitute 1 tablespoon ground flaxseed mixed with 3 tablespoons water for the large egg. Serve these burgers with horseradish and ketchup.

2 teaspoons olive oil
1 medium yellow onion, peeled and chopped
3 cloves garlic, peeled and minced
6 cups chopped fresh baby spinach
1 large egg, beaten
¼ cup chopped walnuts
⅓ cup bread crumbs
3 tablespoons nutritional yeast
1 tablespoon low-sodium soy sauce
1 tablespoon white whole-wheat flour
2 teaspoons all-purpose seasoning
1 teaspoon Tabasco sauce
¼ teaspoon ground black pepper

1. Preheat oven to 375°F. Line a baking sheet with parchment and set aside.
2. In a large sauté pan, heat oil over medium heat. Add onion and cook, stirring, 2 minutes, until it begins to sweat. Add garlic and spinach and cook, stirring, 3 minutes until wilted. Remove pan from heat and transfer contents to a medium bowl.
3. Add remaining ingredients to bowl and stir well to combine. Scoop mixture out by roughly ¼ cup at a time and form into patties. Mixture will be sticky so wash hands as necessary.
4. Place patties on baking sheet. Place sheet on middle rack in oven and bake 10 minutes. Gently flip patties over and bake another 10 minutes, until firm and lightly golden.
5. Remove from oven and serve immediately.

Serves 6

Per Serving

Calories	111
Fat	6g
Protein	5g
Sodium	626mg
Fiber	2g
Carbohydrates	10g
Sugar	2g

Eat Your Spinach!

Spinach is low in calories, high in fiber and protein, and an excellent source of vitamins A, B_6, C, E, and K. Just one serving of spinach a day has been shown to slow cognitive decline. It's delicious in both savory dishes as well as sweet drinks, like fruit smoothies, making it a great addition to almost any meal. Other ways to incorporate more spinach into your diet: Instead of lettuce in your sandwiches substitute fresh baby spinach; or chop and stir into soups, stews, curries, or pilafs for an added burst of nutrients.

Homemade Black Bean Burgers

The combination of nuts, beans, and vital wheat gluten gives these burgers a heft and chew that's irresistible. Substitute any type of unsalted nuts or sunflower seeds for the walnuts if desired. Instead of oven baking, these burgers may also be pan-fried in olive oil on the stovetop.

Serves 4

Per Serving

Calories	434
Fat	12g
Protein	30g
Sodium	1,494mg
Fiber	13g
Carbohydrates	55g
Sugar	6g

What Is Vital Wheat Gluten?

Gluten is the natural protein found in wheat. It's what gives bread its beloved dense chew. Vital wheat gluten is the powdered form of this gluten—basically wheat protein in a box—which can be added to breads and other recipes to make them chewier. It's sold in the baking aisle of most supermarkets, alongside the flour and sugar, and in many natural food stores. Vital wheat gluten looks like flour, and feels like flour, but once it's incorporated with liquids, it becomes so much more.

½ cup chopped walnuts

1 (15-ounce) can black beans, drained and rinsed

1 small yellow onion, peeled and quartered

2 tablespoons low-sodium soy sauce

2 teaspoons all-purpose seasoning

1 teaspoon ground paprika

¼ teaspoon ground black pepper

⅓ cup vital wheat gluten

4 whole-grain hamburger rolls

1 medium tomato, sliced

¼ small red onion, peeled and thinly sliced

1 ounce baby arugula

1. Place walnuts in a food processor and pulse until finely chopped.
2. Add beans, yellow onion, soy sauce, seasoning, paprika, and pepper and pulse until smooth.
3. Add wheat gluten and process until mixture comes together to form a firm dough. The mixture should gather up and spin as a cohesive ball. Test the firmness with a fingertip. If dough is still sticky or isn't coming together well, add additional wheat gluten 1–2 tablespoons at a time until it firms up and is easy to handle.
4. Remove firm dough from food processor and roll into a tight ball. Place on clean surface and cut in half, then half again, to form 4 equal wedges. Roll each wedge into a ball, then press to form a patty.
5. Preheat oven to 350°F. Line a baking sheet with parchment.
6. Arrange patties on baking sheet several inches apart. Place sheet on middle rack in oven and bake 12–15 minutes. Then flip patties and bake another 12–15 minutes. To achieve a crisper crust, spray or brush the burgers lightly with olive oil before baking.
7. Place burgers on rolls and top with tomato, red onion, and arugula. Serve immediately.

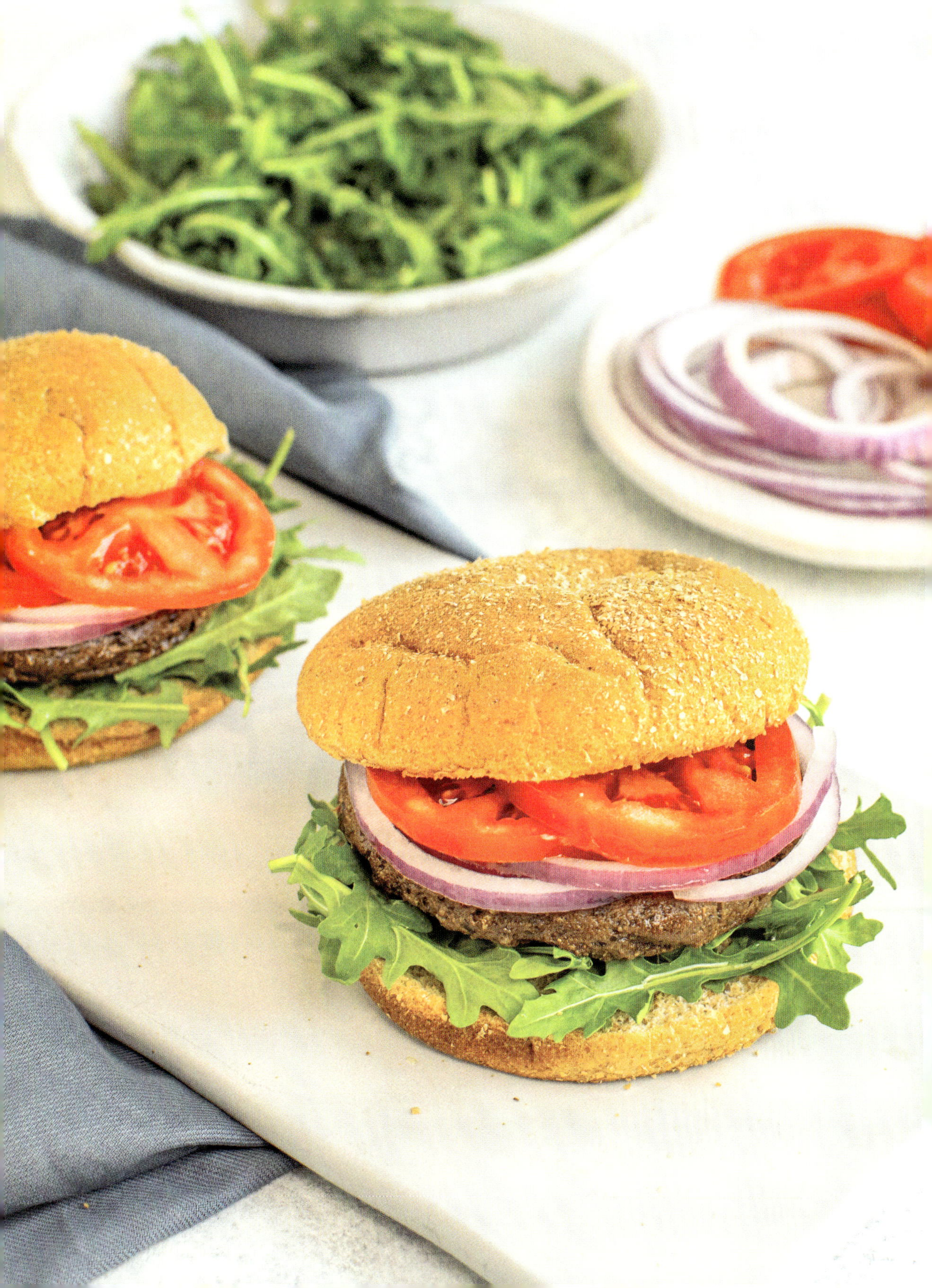

Peanut Butter Noodles

This noodle dish is quick, easy, inexpensive, and perfect for busy weeknight dinners. It comes together as quickly as you can cook the pasta and can be bulked up with whatever sautéed vegetables or dark leafy greens you have on hand. If you don't have tahini, add an extra tablespoon of peanut butter.

Serves 6

Per Serving

Calories	259
Fat	6g
Protein	10g
Sodium	257mg
Fiber	7g
Carbohydrates	43g
Sugar	4g

1 (12-ounce) package whole-grain spaghetti
1 cup vegetable broth
1 tablespoon apple cider vinegar
1½ tablespoons low-sodium soy sauce
3 tablespoons creamy natural peanut butter
1 tablespoon tahini
2 cloves garlic, peeled and minced
2 teaspoons agave nectar
1½ teaspoons Tabasco sauce
½ cup chopped fresh cilantro
⅛ teaspoon ground black pepper

1. Cook spaghetti according to package directions.
2. In a small saucepan add broth, vinegar, soy sauce, peanut butter, tahini, garlic, agave, and Tabasco. Place over low heat and whisk until smooth. Remove from heat.
3. Drain pasta and return to pot. Pour sauce over pasta using a spatula to scrape everything out of the saucepan. Add cilantro and pepper to pot and toss for a minute to coat pasta completely. Serve immediately.

Slow Cooker Cilantro, Potato, and Pea Curry

This dish is made up of tender potatoes and peas simmered in a delicious coconut-scented tomato broth. Serve this over cooked brown rice for an extra-hearty, healthy meal. You can substitute vegetable broth for the vegetable juice called for in this recipe.

1 large yellow onion, peeled and diced
6 cloves garlic, peeled and minced
2 cups vegetable juice
1 (13.5-ounce) can light coconut milk
6 tablespoons tomato paste
8 medium potatoes, peeled and cut into 1" cubes
3 cups fresh or frozen green peas
2 tablespoons low-sodium soy sauce
2 tablespoons unflavored rice wine vinegar
2 tablespoons curry powder
1 tablespoon agave nectar
1 teaspoon ground ginger
¼ teaspoon ground black pepper
⅓ cup chopped fresh cilantro

1. Place all ingredients except cilantro in a slow cooker. Stir well to combine, cover, and cook on high 6 hours.
2. Stir in cilantro and serve immediately.

Serves 8

Per Serving

Calories	260
Fat	3g
Protein	7g
Sodium	375mg
Fiber	6g
Carbohydrates	51g
Sugar	10g

Curry Powder's Main Ingredient: Turmeric

Turmeric is made from the ground root of the turmeric plant. Its bright yellow color and distinct flavor are used in many types of food, from Indian curries and curry powder to classic American prepared mustard. Turmeric has a slightly bitter taste that works well in combination with other seasonings. It contains manganese and iron and may help reduce the risk of certain types of cancer.

Spicy Pan-Roasted Chickpeas with Tahini Sauce

Addictively delicious, these highly seasoned chickpeas are served atop fresh greens and drizzled with a tangy tahini dressing. Chopped kale, baby spinach, or arugula may be substituted for (or added to) the salad greens if desired.

Serves 6

Per Serving

Calories	234
Fat	11g
Protein	9g
Sodium	259mg
Fiber	8g
Carbohydrates	26g
Sugar	5g

¼ cup tahini

3 tablespoons water

3½ tablespoons lemon juice, divided

2 tablespoons olive oil, divided

1 tablespoon unflavored rice wine vinegar

2 teaspoons low-sodium soy sauce, divided

2 cloves garlic, peeled and minced

2 (15-ounce) cans chickpeas, drained and rinsed

1 teaspoon agave nectar

2 teaspoons ground paprika

2 teaspoons ground cumin

1 teaspoon garlic powder

¼ teaspoon ground cayenne

⅛ teaspoon ground black pepper

6 cups fresh spring mix salad greens

1. Make the dressing: In a small bowl, add tahini, water, 1½ tablespoons lemon juice, 1 tablespoon oil, vinegar, 1 teaspoon soy sauce, and garlic. Whisk well to combine. Set aside. Sauce may be made ahead and refrigerated until serving.
2. In a large sauté pan, heat remaining 1 tablespoon oil over medium-high heat. Add chickpeas and cook, stirring, 5 minutes, until they begin to sizzle. Add remaining 2 tablespoons lemon juice, remaining 1 teaspoon soy sauce, agave, paprika, cumin, garlic powder, cayenne, and pepper and cook, stirring, 1 minute, until coated and tender. Remove pan from heat.
3. Place greens on a serving platter or six plates. Spoon chickpeas over greens and drizzle with tahini dressing. Serve immediately.

Vegetable Casserole with Tofu Topping

This recipe makes great use of carrots, onions, cabbage, and kale. Best of all, they're abundantly available year-round. Sandwiched under a crust of crumbled tofu, bread crumbs, and chopped nuts, this dish is an incredible casserole with tons of taste and texture.

- 3 tablespoons olive oil, divided
- 2 medium yellow onions, peeled and thinly sliced
- ½ medium head green cabbage, sliced
- 1 pound chopped fresh kale leaves
- 3 medium carrots, peeled and sliced into thin sticks
- ½ cup vegetable broth
- 2 tablespoons low-sodium soy sauce
- 1½ cups bread crumbs
- 8 ounces extra-firm tofu, drained
- ¼ cup chopped walnuts
- 3 cloves garlic, peeled
- 2 tablespoons nutritional yeast
- 2 teaspoons dried basil
- 1½ teaspoons dried oregano
- 1 teaspoon ground paprika
- ¼ teaspoon ground black pepper

1. Preheat oven to 350°F. Get out a 9" × 13" oven-safe baking dish and set aside.
2. In a large skillet or sauté pan, heat 1 tablespoon oil over medium heat. Add onions and cook, stirring, until softened, 3 minutes. Add cabbage, kale, carrots, broth, and soy sauce. Skillet will be very full; volume will reduce as vegetables cook. Cover pan and cook, stirring occasionally, until vegetables are just tender, 12 minutes. Transfer contents to baking dish and set aside.
3. To make the topping: In a food processor, add remaining 2 tablespoons oil, bread crumbs, tofu, walnuts, garlic, nutritional yeast, basil, oregano, paprika, and pepper and pulse to combine. Alternatively, mash ingredients together in a large bowl with a potato masher.
4. Sprinkle topping mixture over vegetables in baking dish. Place dish on middle rack in oven and bake uncovered until topping is golden brown and vegetables are heated through, 15–20 minutes.
5. Remove from oven and serve immediately.

Serves 8

Per Serving

Calories	259
Fat	10g
Protein	11g
Sodium	357mg
Fiber	7g
Carbohydrates	31g
Sugar	7g

Walnut Facts

Walnuts are rich in polyunsaturated fats and omega-3 fatty acids, manganese, and copper, and they have been shown to prevent cardiovascular disease, lower cholesterol, and protect against certain types of cancer. Most importantly on the MIND diet, walnuts have been proven to aid in memory retention and strengthen motor development.

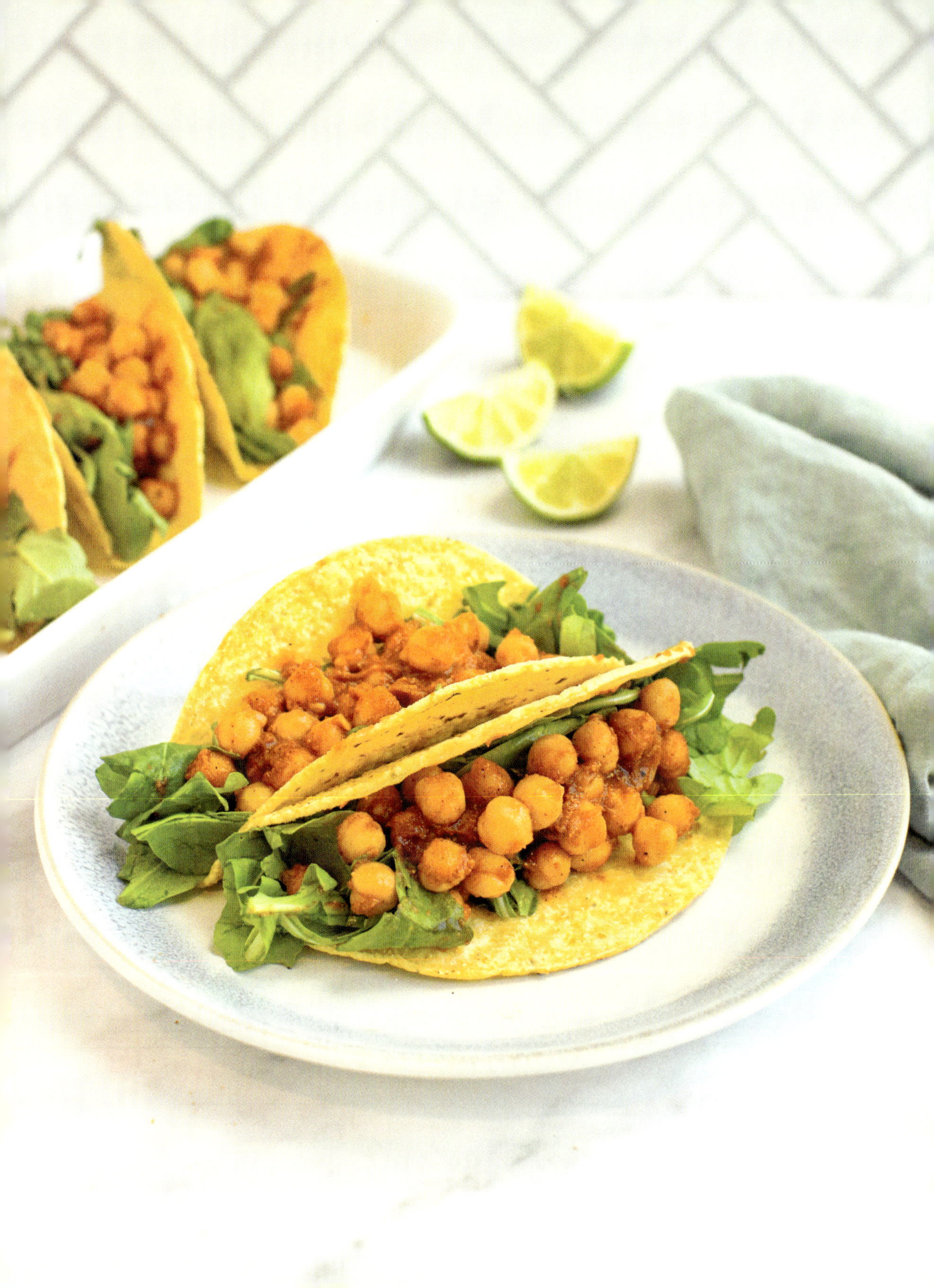

Spicy Chickpea Tacos with Arugula

These tacos feature a thick and spicy tomato-based sauce dotted with chickpeas, the peppery cool of arugula, and the crunchy bite of corn taco shells. Feel free to spoon any extra filling over tortilla chips or cooked brown rice if you run short of shells. For spicier tacos, increase the amount of pepper and pepper flakes.

Serves 6

Per Serving

Calories	268
Fat	7g
Protein	9g
Sodium	384mg
Fiber	8g
Carbohydrates	42g
Sugar	8g

1 (12-count) package corn taco shells

2 (15-ounce) cans chickpeas, drained and rinsed

¼ cup tomato paste

1 tablespoon apple cider vinegar

1 tablespoon light brown sugar

2 teaspoons chili seasoning

1 teaspoon ground mustard

1 teaspoon onion powder

½ teaspoon garlic powder

¼ teaspoon ground black pepper

⅛ teaspoon dried red pepper flakes

6 cups fresh arugula

1. Heat taco shells according to package directions.
2. In a large saucepan, add chickpeas, tomato paste, vinegar, sugar, chili seasoning, mustard, onion powder, garlic powder, black pepper, and red pepper and stir well to combine.
3. Place pan over medium heat and simmer, stirring frequently, 10 minutes.
4. Remove pan from heat. Fill warm taco shells with arugula and then spoon chickpea mixture over top. Serve immediately.

Lemon Pesto Rice with Portobello Mushrooms

This recipe gives you a hearty vegan one-dish meal perfect for weeknights and potluck parties. The bright bite of lemon pesto is fabulous on its own, but partnered with sautéed onion, meaty mushrooms, and brown rice, it's downright addictive. For the pesto, use your favorite type of unsalted nuts: walnuts, pecans, almonds, or cashews.

Serves 6

Per Serving

Calories	354
Fat	11g
Protein	9g
Sodium	247mg
Fiber	5g
Carbohydrates	56g
Sugar	4g

For Fun and Freshness, Grow Your Own!

Fresh herbs are easy and inexpensive to grow in almost any living situation. A sunny windowsill or patio planter can produce enough herbs to flavor a wide array of recipes any time of year. A few pots, some soil, and seeds are all you need to get started.

2½ tablespoons olive oil, divided

1 large yellow onion, peeled and chopped

16 ounces fresh baby bella mushrooms, chopped

6 cups cooked brown rice

Juice of 2 medium lemons

6 cloves garlic, peeled

1½ teaspoons agave nectar

½ teaspoon yellow mustard

⅓ cup chopped walnuts

⅓ cup (packed) fresh basil leaves

2 tablespoons nutritional yeast

1 teaspoon all-purpose seasoning

¼ teaspoon ground black pepper

1. In a large stockpot, heat 1 tablespoon oil over medium heat. Add onion and mushrooms and cook, stirring, 10 minutes, until tender. Remove from heat, stir in cooked rice, cover, and set aside.
2. In a food processor, add remaining 1½ tablespoons oil, lemon juice, garlic, agave, mustard, nuts, basil, nutritional yeast, seasoning, and pepper and pulse until smooth.
3. Stir pesto into rice mixture until well combined. Serve immediately.

Samosa Pasta

In this dish, whole-grain spaghetti is tossed with diced potato and green peas and coated in a flavorful curry sauce. It's like a healthy bowl of samosas in less than 30 minutes!

- 1 (12-ounce) package whole-grain spaghetti
- 2 medium potatoes, scrubbed and pierced with a fork
- 1 tablespoon olive oil
- 1 medium yellow onion, peeled and chopped
- 3 cloves garlic, peeled and minced
- 1 cup frozen green peas, thawed
- 1 cup vegetable broth
- 2 tablespoons apple cider vinegar
- 1½ tablespoons low-sodium soy sauce
- 1 teaspoon agave nectar
- 3 tablespoons nutritional yeast
- 2 teaspoons curry powder
- 1 teaspoon all-purpose seasoning
- 1 teaspoon ground paprika
- ¼ teaspoon dried red pepper flakes
- ⅛ teaspoon ground black pepper
- ¼ cup chopped fresh cilantro

Serves 6

Per Serving

Calories	293
Fat	3g
Protein	12g
Sodium	513mg
Fiber	10g
Carbohydrates	58g
Sugar	5g

1. Cook pasta according to package directions.
2. Place potatoes in microwave and cook 4 minutes on high, then turn them over and cook another 4 minutes. Insert a paring knife into the potatoes to check for doneness. If knife slides in smoothly, potato is done; if not, microwave in 30-second increments until done. Remove potatoes from microwave, let rest briefly to cool, then dice.
3. In a large skillet or sauté pan, heat oil over medium heat. Add onion and sauté 2 minutes, until it begins to sweat. Add garlic and peas and cook, stirring, 1 minute. Add broth and other remaining ingredients except cilantro and cook, stirring, until sauce has thickened slightly, 3–4 minutes.
4. Drain pasta and return to pot. Add potatoes. Pour sauce over top, add cilantro, and toss well to combine. Serve immediately.

Tasty Lentil Tacos

This recipe gives you a speedy and inexpensive MIND diet–appropriate meal. Cooked lentils are soft and brown, with a look and texture not unlike ground beef, and they make an amazing taco filling. Substitute soft taco shells for the crunchy and a spicier salsa for the mild if desired.

Serves 6

Per Serving

Calories	272
Fat	6g
Protein	10g
Sodium	771mg
Fiber	7g
Carbohydrates	43g
Sugar	5g

1 teaspoon olive oil

1 medium yellow onion, peeled and diced

2 garlic cloves, peeled and minced

1 cup uncooked lentils, rinsed

1 tablespoon chili seasoning

2 teaspoons ground cumin

1 teaspoon dried oregano

2½ cups vegetable broth

1 (12-count) package crunchy taco shells

1 cup mild salsa

1. In a large skillet or sauté pan, heat oil over medium heat. Add onion and garlic and cook, stirring, 3 minutes. Add lentils, chili seasoning, cumin, and oregano and cook, stirring, 1 minute, until fragrant.
2. Add broth and bring to a boil over high heat; then reduce heat to low, cover, and simmer 30 minutes.
3. Warm taco shells according to directions on package.
4. Remove lentils from heat, uncover pan, and mash lentils slightly. Stir in salsa.
5. Spoon roughly ¼ cup filling into each taco shell and serve immediately.

Meatless Meatloaf

This recipe is melt-in-your-mouth comfort food. If you are looking for condiments to serve with this that are more in line with the MIND diet principles, recipes for homemade ketchup, barbecue sauce, and honey mustard are in Chapter 5.

- 3 teaspoons olive oil, divided
- 3 medium potatoes, scrubbed and cubed
- 1 (15-ounce) can kidney beans, drained and rinsed
- 1 medium red bell pepper, seeded and chopped
- 1 medium yellow onion, peeled and chopped
- 3 cloves garlic, peeled and minced
- 2 teaspoons ground cumin
- 1 teaspoon chili seasoning
- 1½ cups quick oats
- ½ cup barbecue sauce, divided
- ¼ cup ketchup
- 2½ teaspoons yellow mustard
- ½ teaspoon ground black pepper
- ¼ cup chopped fresh cilantro
- 2 tablespoons nutritional yeast

Serves 6

Per Serving

Calories	309
Fat	4g
Protein	10g
Sodium	483mg
Fiber	9g
Carbohydrates	59g
Sugar	13g

1. Preheat oven to 375°F. Lightly oil an 8" square baking pan with 1 teaspoon oil and set aside.
2. Place potatoes in a large saucepan. Add enough water to cover, bring to a boil over high heat, then reduce heat slightly and cook until tender, roughly 15 minutes. Drain and mash potatoes. Set aside.
3. In a medium bowl, mash beans using the tines of a fork and set aside.
4. In a large skillet, heat remaining 2 teaspoons oil over medium heat. Add bell pepper, onion, garlic, cumin, and chili seasoning and cook, stirring, 3 minutes, until they begin to sweat. Remove from heat. Stir in potatoes, beans, oats, ¼ cup barbecue sauce, ketchup, mustard, black pepper, and cilantro.
5. Spoon mixture into prepared pan and smooth top to even. Spread remaining ¼ cup barbecue sauce over top and sprinkle with nutritional yeast.
6. Place pan on middle rack in oven and bake 35 minutes, until hot and steaming. Remove from oven, let rest 10 minutes, slice, and serve warm.

Chana Masala

In this version of the traditional Indian dish, chickpeas, tomatoes, and greens are simmered in a spicy, seasoned sauce. Serve this dish over cooked brown rice for a super satisfying meal. Swiss chard, baby kale, or spinach may be substituted for the collard greens if desired.

Serves 4

Per Serving

Calories	234
Fat	2g
Protein	11g
Sodium	598mg
Fiber	11g
Carbohydrates	41g
Sugar	10g

What Is Garam Masala?

Garam masala is a ground spice blend used extensively in Indian cooking. Though blends may differ, garam masala typically includes cinnamon, cumin, coriander, cloves, ginger, nutmeg, pepper, mace, star anise, and bay leaves. Garam masala is potent in terms of fragrance and flavor, but unlike many curry powders, it does not tend to be fiery hot.

1½ cups vegetable broth, divided

1 medium yellow onion, peeled and diced

3 cloves garlic, peeled and minced

1 medium jalapeño pepper, seeded and minced

1 teaspoon curry powder

½ teaspoon garam masala

¼ teaspoon ground ginger

1 (14.5-ounce) can no-salt-added diced tomatoes, with juice

2 (15-ounce) cans chickpeas, drained and rinsed

4 cups chopped fresh collard greens, stems removed

¼ cup chopped fresh cilantro

1 tablespoon lemon juice

1. In a large sauté pan, heat ½ cup broth over medium-high heat. Add onion, garlic, and jalapeño and cook, stirring, 5 minutes.
2. Add curry powder, garam masala, and ginger and stir until fragrant. Add tomatoes, chickpeas, and remaining 1 cup broth and bring to a simmer. Reduce heat to medium and cook, stirring frequently, 15 minutes.
3. Add collard greens, cover, and cook until tender, stirring occasionally, 10 minutes.
4. Remove from heat. Add cilantro and lemon juice and stir to combine. Serve immediately.

CHAPTER 8

Vegetables and Sides

Sweet and Spicy Brussels Sprouts

Spicy, sweet, tangy, and irresistible, the combination of flavors in these Sweet and Spicy Brussels Sprouts will keep you reaching for more. Feel free to double the recipe, but even then, you may not get enough!

Serves 8

Per Serving

Calories	60
Fat	2g
Protein	3g
Sodium	112mg
Fiber	3g
Carbohydrates	10g
Sugar	4g

2 pounds Brussels sprouts, trimmed and larger ones halved

1 tablespoon agave nectar

1 tablespoon lime juice

1 tablespoon low-sodium soy sauce

1 tablespoon olive oil

1 tablespoon sriracha

½ teaspoon ground black pepper

1. Preheat oven to 400°F. Line a baking sheet with parchment and set aside.
2. Place Brussels sprouts in a medium bowl.
3. In a small bowl, add agave, lime juice, soy sauce, oil, and sriracha and whisk well to combine. Pour mixture over Brussels sprouts and toss well to coat.
4. Spread Brussels sprouts in a single layer on the parchment and sprinkle with pepper. Place baking sheet on middle rack in oven and bake 35 minutes until tender.
5. Remove sheet from oven. Serve immediately.

Sriracha Facts

Sriracha is a spicy red chili sauce made from chili peppers, distilled vinegar, garlic, sugar, and salt. Originally from Thailand, it's become one of the most popular condiments in the world. Even a tiny bit will add a lot of flavor, not to mention heat, to many dishes. Look for it in the Asian section of most supermarkets. It's sold under several name brands; a top seller is Huy Fong, which has a rooster on the bottle.

Perfect Steamed Broccoli

Here's a foolproof recipe for making perfectly crisp, perfectly seasoned broccoli every time. In this recipe the broccoli is steamed gently in a small amount of vegetable broth instead of plain water. The flavor of the broth permeates the spears, leaving them tasty and tender.

½ cup vegetable broth

1½ pounds fresh broccoli spears

½ teaspoon ground black pepper

1. Place a medium stockpot over medium-high heat. Add broth and then place a steamer basket inside pot. Arrange broccoli evenly in the steamer. Cover pan and set a kitchen timer to 7 minutes.
2. Stir broccoli once or twice while cooking, then check spears after 7 minutes for doneness. If tender, remove from heat immediately. If still a bit too crisp, cover pot and check every minute; cook no more than 10 minutes total.
3. Remove from heat and sprinkle with pepper. Serve immediately.

Serves 4

Per Serving

Calories	58
Fat	0g
Protein	5g
Sodium	56mg
Fiber	5g
Carbohydrates	12g
Sugar	3g

Five-Spice Fried Rice

The key to making perfect fried rice is to use cold rice only—so this is a great way to use up leftover rice. Make this recipe as written or use whatever protein and vegetables you have on hand. Serve with chopped cashews or peanuts and sliced scallions.

Serves 6

Per Serving

Calories	199
Fat	3g
Protein	5g
Sodium	165mg
Fiber	4g
Carbohydrates	39g
Sugar	3g

2 teaspoons olive oil
1 medium yellow onion, peeled and diced
3 cloves garlic, peeled and minced
2 medium carrots, peeled and diced
4 cups cold cooked brown rice
1 cup frozen green peas
1½ tablespoons low-sodium soy sauce
1 tablespoon unflavored rice wine vinegar
1 teaspoon sriracha
½ teaspoon ground ginger
¼ teaspoon five-spice powder
½ teaspoon ground black pepper

1. In a wok or large sauté pan, heat oil over medium heat. Add onion, garlic, and carrots and cook, stirring, 5 minutes.
2. Add remaining ingredients and stir well to coat. Cook, stirring, 5 minutes until rice is fragrant and vegetables are tender.
3. Remove from heat and serve immediately.

Make Your Own Five-Spice Powder

To make your own five-spice powder: Combine 1 teaspoon ground cinnamon, 1 teaspoon anise seed or 1 star anise, ¼ teaspoon fennel seeds, ¼ teaspoon ground black pepper, and ⅛ teaspoon ground cloves. Grind into a powder using a small spice grinder or mortar and pestle. This yields 1 tablespoon; you only need ¼ teaspoon for this recipe. Sealed in a clean, lidded jar or plastic bag, the excess spice mixture should remain fresh for 2 years.

Roasted Lemon Asparagus

In this recipe, fresh asparagus is tossed with lemon juice and a tiny bit of oil, then oven roasted. What sounds so simple becomes an extraordinarily delicious side dish, full of citrus flavor and complexity.

1½ pounds fresh asparagus, trimmed and cut into 3" pieces

2 tablespoons lemon juice

1 teaspoon olive oil

½ teaspoon ground black pepper

1. Preheat oven to 425°F. Line a baking sheet with parchment and set aside.
2. In a medium bowl, add asparagus, lemon juice, oil, and pepper. Toss gently to coat.
3. Spread asparagus in a single layer on baking sheet. Place sheet on middle rack in oven and roast until tender, 20 minutes.
4. Remove from oven. Serve immediately.

Serves 6

Per Serving

Calories	22
Fat	1g
Protein	2g
Sodium	1mg
Fiber	2g
Carbohydrates	3g
Sugar	2g

Roasting for Flavor

Roasting is simply cooking food at a very high temperature. Oven roasting allows for convenience and control, as you're able to adjust not only the temperature of the oven but the proximity of the food to the flame. The roasting process allows the natural sugars present in many foods to caramelize, leaving the cooked versions much sweeter and more complex than they were when raw.

Swiss Chard with Apples, Raisins, and Pecans

In this recipe the sweetness of the apples and raisins tempers the bitterness of the greens, rendering them addictively delicious. For variety, you can substitute kale or beet greens for the chard, and walnuts and dried cranberries for the pecans and raisins.

Serves 8

Per Serving

Calories	136
Fat	8g
Protein	2g
Sodium	187mg
Fiber	3g
Carbohydrates	15g
Sugar	10g

Swiss Chard Facts

Swiss chard is a dark leafy green with colorful stalks akin to celery. It has a somewhat bitter taste that mellows with cooking and is particularly well suited to sautéing with a little olive oil and garlic. Swiss chard is an excellent source of vitamins A, C, and K, plus manganese, potassium, iron, fiber, and antioxidants, and it has been linked to the prevention of Alzheimer's, cancer, and cardiovascular disease.

½ cup water

¼ cup seedless raisins

2 tablespoons olive oil

1 medium red onion, peeled and diced

1½ pounds fresh Swiss chard, stems removed and sliced, leaves chopped

2 large Honeycrisp apples, peeled, cored, and diced

½ cup chopped pecans

1 tablespoon low-sodium soy sauce

1 tablespoon apple cider vinegar

2 teaspoons agave nectar

½ teaspoon ground black pepper

1. Place water in a kettle, microwave-safe bowl, or small saucepan and heat until boiling.
2. Place raisins in a small bowl and add boiling water to cover. Set aside to plump.
3. In a large sauté pan over medium heat, warm oil. Add onion and cook, stirring, 2 minutes. Add chard stems and apples and cook, stirring, 2 minutes, until they begin to sweat.
4. Drain raisins but reserve 1 tablespoon soaking water. Add raisins and reserved water to pan along with chard leaves and stir well to combine. Cover pan and cook 6 minutes until chard is wilted and tender.
5. Uncover pan and stir briefly to release any extra liquid. Add remaining ingredients and stir well to combine.
6. Remove from heat and serve immediately.

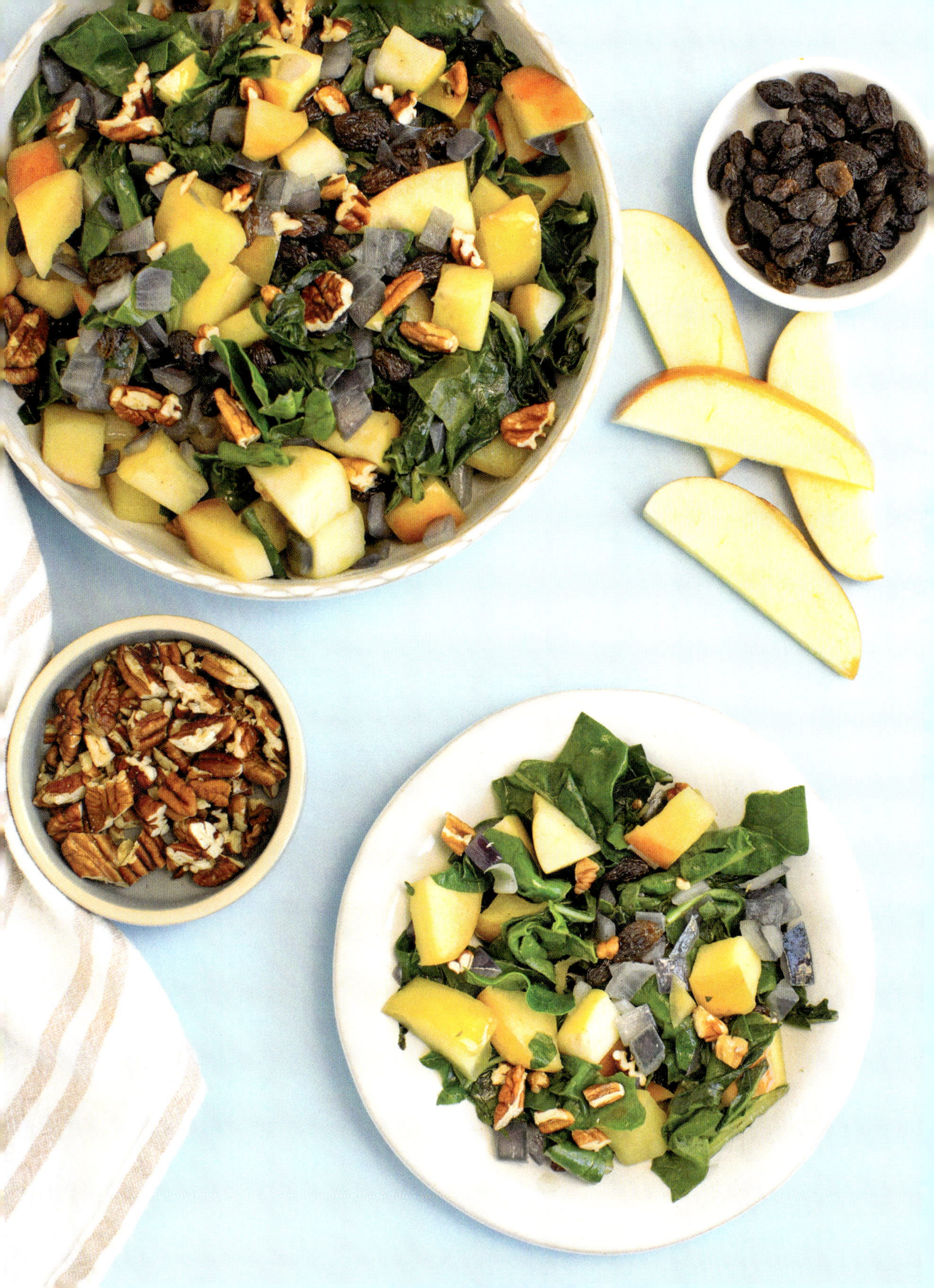

Butternut Squash with Brown Sugar and Walnuts

Here, the natural sweetness of butternut squash is heightened with brown sugar and cinnamon. The flavor pairs wonderfully with poultry, making this an ideal side for the holidays. For a twist on the same dish, use sweet potatoes and pecans and reduce the cooking time by 10 minutes.

Serves 6

Per Serving

Calories	131
Fat	3g
Protein	2g
Sodium	8mg
Fiber	3g
Carbohydrates	27g
Sugar	12g

6 cups cubed butternut squash

1 tablespoon olive oil

¼ cup (unpacked) dark brown sugar

¼ cup chopped walnuts

1 teaspoon ground cinnamon

1. Preheat oven to 425°F. Line a baking sheet with parchment and set aside.
2. In a large bowl, add squash, oil, sugar, walnuts, and cinnamon and toss well to coat.
3. Arrange squash on baking sheet. Place sheet on middle rack in oven and bake until tender, 45 minutes.
4. Remove from oven and serve immediately.

Oven-Baked Sweet Potato Fries

These versatile potato wedges can be served with a myriad of main courses. You can vary the flavor of the seasoning: Southwestern, lemon-pepper, all-purpose, Jamaican jerk, and so on. For a sweeter version, toss with 2 tablespoons brown sugar and ½ teaspoon ground cinnamon.

4 medium sweet potatoes, peeled and cut into wedges

1 tablespoon olive oil

1 teaspoon all-purpose seasoning

½ teaspoon ground black pepper

1. Preheat oven to 425°F. Line a baking sheet with parchment and set aside.
2. In a large bowl, add sweet potatoes, oil, seasoning, and pepper and toss well to coat.
3. Arrange wedges on baking sheet. Place on middle rack in oven and bake 20 minutes. Flip wedges, then return to oven and bake another 15 minutes until tender.
4. Remove from oven and serve immediately.

Serves 4

Per Serving

Calories	103
Fat	0g
Protein	2g
Sodium	391mg
Fiber	4g
Carbohydrates	24g
Sugar	8g

Sweet Potato Facts

Sweet potatoes are a staple anyone on the MIND diet should embrace. They're high in vitamins A, B_6, and C; they contain beta-carotene, magnesium, calcium, iron, protein, and fiber; and they are low in sodium. When buying sweet potatoes, look for firm orange flesh, free of soft spots or blemishes. At home, store them in a dark cabinet or drawer, never in the refrigerator.

Baked Spinach and Pea Risotto

There's something magical about the combination of tastes and textures in this risotto. Vegans can eliminate the cheese altogether—the risotto will be just as delicious without it. If you're looking to replace the wine, substitute ¼ cup vegetable broth plus 2–3 tablespoons white wine vinegar.

Serves 6

Per Serving

Calories	193
Fat	3g
Protein	5g
Sodium	507mg
Fiber	1g
Carbohydrates	33g
Sugar	3g

Hidden Substances in Frozen Vegetables

Many frozen vegetables are just that, frozen vegetables. But others contain things you don't want, like added salt and sauces. When selecting frozen vegetables, check nutrition facts carefully to ensure you're buying the vegetables you want, without anything else.

1 tablespoon olive oil

1 medium shallot, peeled and chopped

½ teaspoon ground black pepper

½ cup dry white wine

3 cups vegetable broth

1 cup uncooked Arborio rice

1 cup frozen green peas, thawed

2 cups chopped fresh baby spinach

¼ cup grated Parmesan cheese

1. Preheat oven to 425°F.
2. Place a Dutch oven (or similar oven-safe lidded pot) on the stovetop over medium-high heat. Add oil, shallot, and pepper and sauté 3 minutes.
3. Add wine and cook, stirring, until almost evaporated, 2 minutes.
4. Stir in broth and rice and bring to a boil, then cover pot and transfer to middle rack in oven. Bake 20 minutes until rice is tender and creamy.
5. Remove from oven. Add peas, spinach, and cheese and stir well to combine. Serve immediately.

Garlicky Green Beans

This dish is simple enough for you to prepare daily, and you'll never tire of eating these beans, either straight from the pan or on a plate for dinner. For larger parties or holidays, double the recipe, but make the beans a pound at a time; they won't cook perfectly if overcrowded in the pan.

Serves 4

Per Serving

Calories	59
Fat	2g
Protein	2g
Sodium	182mg
Fiber	3g
Carbohydrates	9g
Sugar	4g

1 cup water

1 pound fresh green beans, washed and trimmed

2 teaspoons olive oil

4 cloves garlic, peeled and minced

½ teaspoon all-purpose seasoning

½ teaspoon ground black pepper

1. In a large sauté pan, heat water over medium heat. Add green beans and stir to coat. Cook, stirring frequently, 5 minutes.
2. Remove pan from heat and drain beans into a large colander. Rinse beans under cold water.
3. Return pan to medium heat, add oil and garlic, and cook, stirring, 1–2 minutes. Add beans and cook, stirring, just until tender, 2–3 minutes.
4. Remove from heat and sprinkle with seasoning and pepper. Serve immediately.

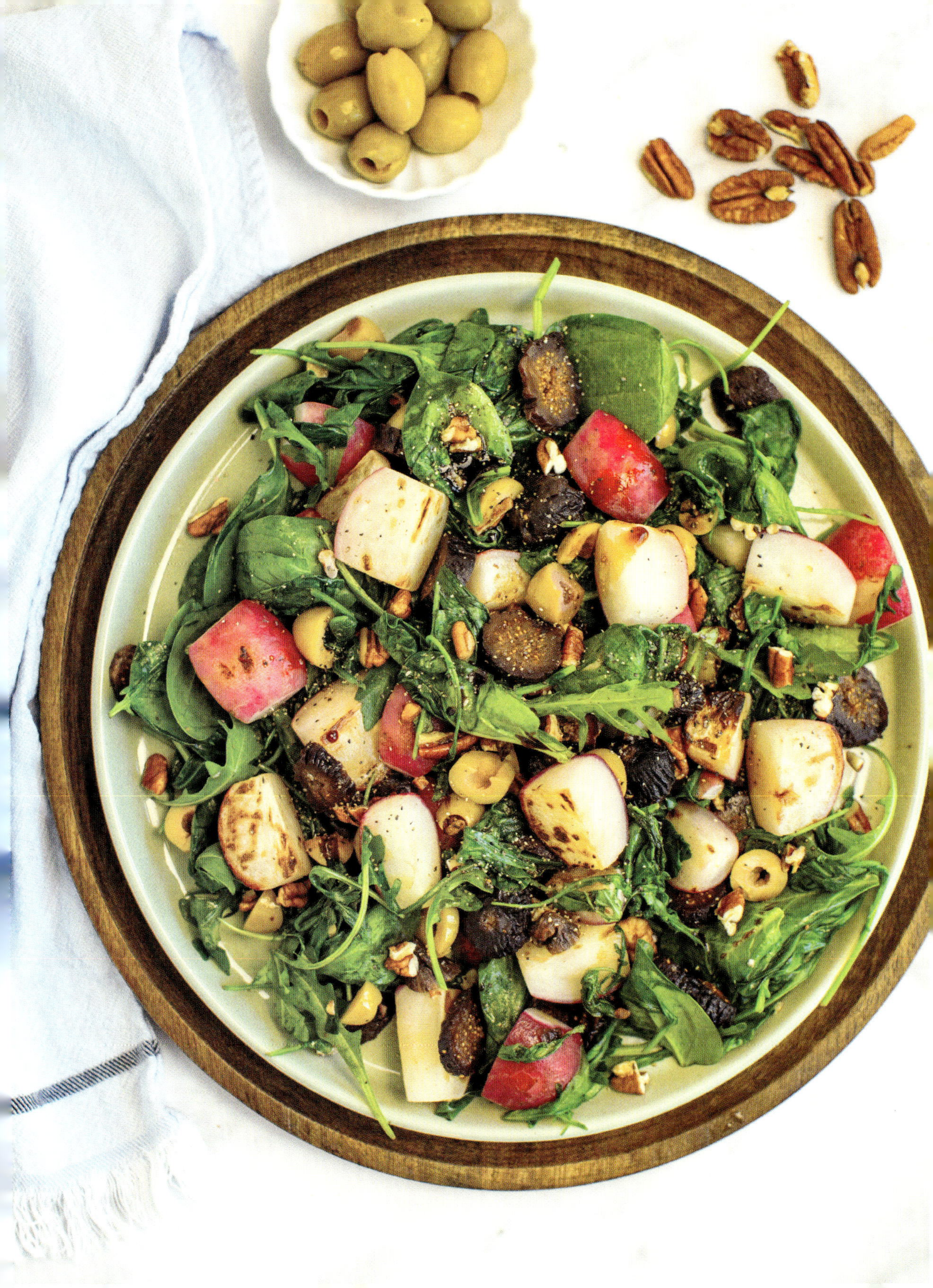

Pan-Roasted Radishes with Figs and Greens

Cooked radishes have a milder flavor than their raw counterparts. Here they're browned until tender, then tossed with plumped figs, pecans, and fresh greens. If you enjoy radish greens, substitute an equal amount for the arugula.

1 cup water
½ cup sliced dried Mission figs
2 tablespoons olive oil, divided
2 cups (10 ounces) trimmed radishes, halved or quartered
8 cups fresh baby spinach
4 cups fresh arugula
¼ cup chopped pecans
¼ cup pitted and chopped green olives
2 teaspoons balsamic vinegar
½ teaspoon ground black pepper

1. Place water in a kettle, microwave-safe bowl, or small saucepan and heat until boiling.
2. Place figs in a small bowl and cover with boiling water. Set aside 5 minutes to plump, then drain.
3. In a large sauté pan over medium-high heat, warm 1 tablespoon oil. Add radishes, cover, and cook undisturbed 3 minutes until brown on one side. Uncover, shake pan, and cook another 3–4 minutes until radishes are tender. Remove from heat, place radishes in a medium bowl, and set aside.
4. Return pan to heat and add the remaining 1 tablespoon oil. Add spinach and arugula and cook while stirring with tongs until barely wilted, about 2 minutes.
5. Add figs, pecans, olives, and radishes. Cover pan and cook 3 minutes until everything is heated through.
6. Remove from heat, uncover, and drizzle with vinegar. Add pepper and serve immediately.

Serves 6

Per Serving

Calories	111
Fat	9g
Protein	2g
Sodium	167mg
Fiber	3g
Carbohydrates	7g
Sugar	4g

Radish Facts

Radishes are a member of the *Brassica* (cabbage) genus and are related to kale, broccoli, and cauliflower. Radishes are a quick and easy-growing crop, perfect for any home garden. All of the plant is edible, both the leaves and root, and can be eaten raw or cooked. Radishes are low in calories and high in vitamin C, antioxidants, minerals, and fiber.

Southwestern Corn Sauté

The perfect partner for taco night, this speedy side might become the star of the show. A can of black or pinto beans easily transforms this into a burrito filling; a can of diced tomatoes makes it an extra-hearty warm salsa for spooning over nachos or serving with tortilla chips. No need to thaw the frozen corn; it cooks fully in the pan.

Serves 6

Per Serving

Calories	131
Fat	5g
Protein	3g
Sodium	13mg
Fiber	4g
Carbohydrates	21g
Sugar	4g

Avocado Facts

Ripe avocados have a smooth, leathery skin that when ripe yields to pressure. The easiest way to prepare a ripe avocado is to cut lengthwise through the fruit to the core, gently break open, remove the pit, and peel away the skin. Avocados are high in vitamins B_6, C, E, and K, and have been shown to protect against prostate cancer.

2 teaspoons olive oil
1 medium red onion, peeled and diced
1 medium green bell pepper, seeded and diced
1 medium red bell pepper, seeded and diced
3 cups frozen corn kernels
3 cloves garlic, peeled and minced
2 tablespoons lime juice
1 teaspoon agave nectar
1 teaspoon ground cumin
½ teaspoon dried oregano
½ teaspoon chili seasoning
⅛ teaspoon ground cayenne
1 medium ripe avocado, peeled, pitted, and diced
¼ cup chopped fresh cilantro
½ teaspoon ground black pepper

1. In a large sauté pan, heat oil over medium heat. Add onion and cook, stirring, 2 minutes.
2. Add green and red peppers and cook, stirring, 3 minutes.
3. Add corn, garlic, lime juice, agave, cumin, oregano, chili seasoning, and cayenne and stir well to combine. Cook, stirring frequently, 5 minutes.
4. Remove from heat. Stir in avocado, cilantro, and black pepper. Serve immediately.

Coconut Quinoa with Kale

Warm, comforting, and filled with flavor, this quinoa "pilaf" is reminiscent of couscous. Even if you think you dislike coconut and quinoa, you may be surprised at how much you enjoy this speedy side! Try it for yourself; it may become a favorite too.

Serves 4

Per Serving

Calories	249
Fat	8g
Protein	7g
Sodium	68mg
Fiber	4g
Carbohydrates	36g
Sugar	3g

1 cup uncooked quinoa

1 (13.5-ounce) can light coconut milk, divided

¼ cup chopped fresh cilantro

1 teaspoon olive oil

1 medium yellow onion, peeled and diced

3 cloves garlic, peeled and minced

4 cups chopped fresh kale leaves

1½ teaspoons agave nectar

1½ teaspoons apple cider vinegar

1½ teaspoons lime juice

1½ teaspoons low-sodium soy sauce

½ teaspoon ground black pepper

1. Place quinoa in a fine-mesh sieve and rinse under cold water for a minute or two. Transfer quinoa to a medium saucepan, add 1 cup coconut milk, and stir to combine.
2. Bring to a boil over medium-high heat; then lower the heat to medium-low, cover, and simmer 15 minutes. Remove from heat, uncover, and fluff quinoa. Add cilantro and toss to combine. Set aside.
3. In a large sauté pan, heat oil over medium heat. Add onion and garlic and cook, stirring, 2 minutes. Add kale, agave, vinegar, lime juice, soy sauce, and remaining coconut milk and stir to combine. Cook, stirring frequently, 8 minutes or until most of the liquid has evaporated.
4. Remove from heat, add quinoa, and stir to combine. Add pepper and serve immediately.

Red Potatoes with Mustard, Peas, and Parsley

Simple peas and potatoes are elevated to new heights in this recipe with the addition of mustard, wine, and onion. You can also add a couple of chopped hard-boiled eggs or a cup of cooked beans for extra protein if desired.

Serves 4

Per Serving

Calories	232
Fat	4g
Protein	6g
Sodium	145mg
Fiber	5g
Carbohydrates	41g
Sugar	5g

1½ pounds red potatoes, scrubbed and cut into 1½" cubes

1 cup frozen green peas

¼ cup dry white wine

1 small yellow onion, peeled and chopped

2 tablespoons yellow mustard

1 tablespoon olive oil

½ teaspoon ground black pepper

¼ cup chopped fresh parsley

1. Place potatoes in a large pot, add enough water to cover by an inch, and bring to a boil over high heat. Boil until tender, about 15 minutes. Add peas to the pot during the last 2–3 minutes of cooking.
2. Drain potatoes and peas into a colander and set aside. Do not wash pot.
3. Return pot to stove, place over high heat, and add wine and onion. Cook 2 minutes to soften, then remove pot from heat and whisk in mustard, oil, and pepper.
4. Add potatoes and peas back into pot and toss well to coat. Add parsley and stir to combine. Serve immediately.

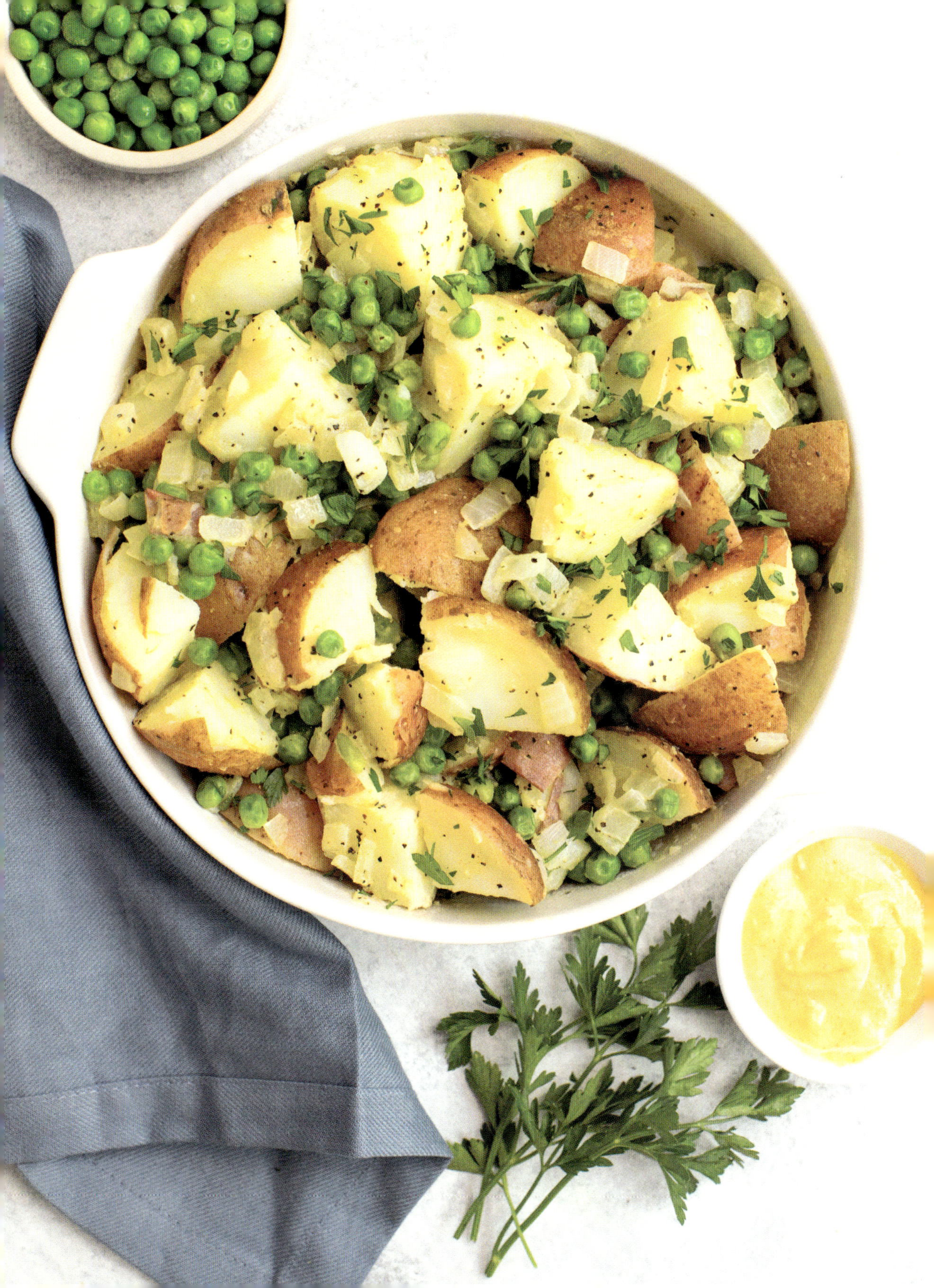

Oven-Roasted Cherry Tomatoes

In this recipe cherry tomatoes are rendered irresistible with little more than some heat. This recipe works wonderfully not only with ripe red tomatoes but with unripe green tomatoes too. You can store leftovers in the refrigerator up to 3 days.

Serves 4

Per Serving

Calories	58
Fat	3g
Protein	1g
Sodium	357mg
Fiber	2g
Carbohydrates	6g
Sugar	4g

The Many Uses of Oven-Roasted Tomatoes

In addition to being eaten plain, roasted tomatoes can be used as a topping for tacos or burritos; as a filling for wrap sandwiches; as a stand-in for canned tomatoes in your favorite soup, stew, or chili; as a base for pasta sauce or salsa verde; and more!

4 cups cherry tomatoes

1 tablespoon olive oil

1 teaspoon all-purpose seasoning

½ teaspoon garlic powder

¼ teaspoon dried thyme

¼ teaspoon ground black pepper

1. Preheat oven to 425°F. Line a rimmed baking sheet with parchment and set aside.
2. In a medium bowl, add all ingredients and toss well to coat.
3. Place tomatoes on baking sheet and roll gently to arrange in a single layer. Place sheet on middle rack in oven and bake 45–60 minutes until tomatoes are nicely deflated and juicy.
4. Remove from oven. Serve hot or cold.

Oven-Baked Mushroom Barley Pilaf

This creamy pilaf filled with the earthy flavors of mushrooms and barley is warm comfort food at its best. Easy serving and wide appeal make this a great potluck dish, especially in the winter, and the hands-off oven baking makes cooking a breeze.

2 tablespoons olive oil

10 ounces fresh mushrooms, chopped

1 medium yellow onion, peeled and chopped

4 cloves garlic, peeled and minced

¼ cup chopped walnuts

½ cup red wine

1 cup uncooked pearl barley

3 cups vegetable broth

1 bay leaf

1 teaspoon all-purpose seasoning

½ teaspoon dried basil

¼ teaspoon dried thyme

¼ teaspoon dried marjoram

¼ teaspoon ground black pepper

¼ cup chopped fresh parsley

1. Preheat oven to 350°F.
2. In a Dutch oven (or similar oven-safe lidded pot), heat oil over medium heat. Add mushrooms, onion, and garlic and cook, stirring, 5 minutes.
3. Add walnuts, wine, barley, broth, bay leaf, seasoning, basil, thyme, marjoram, and pepper and cook, stirring frequently, 5 minutes.
4. Cover pot and transfer to middle rack in oven. Bake 1 hour until barley is tender.
5. Remove from oven. Carefully remove bay leaf and discard. Stir in parsley and serve immediately.

Serves 6

Per Serving

Calories	223
Fat	8g
Protein	6g
Sodium	641mg
Fiber	7g
Carbohydrates	32g
Sugar	3g

Mushroom Facts

Mushrooms are extremely low in fat and calories, and are a great source of copper, selenium, B vitamins, and antioxidants. Mushrooms have been shown to boost immunity against infection, inhibit cancer, reduce inflammation, and protect against cardiovascular and other diseases. At home, store fresh mushrooms in the refrigerator; the cold inhibits discoloration and helps maintain their phytonutrient content.

Roasted Beets with Chili Lime Vinaigrette

This delicious side will appeal to even the staunchest of beet haters. The natural sweetness of the beets is accentuated by oven roasting; the tender beets are then tossed with ripe orange, mango, and almonds and drizzled with a stellar spicy-citrus vinaigrette.

Serves 4

Per Serving

Calories	235
Fat	14g
Protein	4g
Sodium	81mg
Fiber	5g
Carbohydrates	27g
Sugar	20g

2 medium beets, trimmed and washed
4 cups fresh mixed salad greens
1 large orange, peeled and cut into bite-sized chunks
1 medium mango, peeled, cored, and diced
¼ cup slivered almonds
3 tablespoons lime juice
1 tablespoon apple cider vinegar
2 teaspoons agave nectar
3 tablespoons olive oil
1 teaspoon yellow mustard
1 teaspoon ground cumin
½ teaspoon chili seasoning

1. Preheat oven to 400°F.
2. Wrap beets tightly in aluminum foil. Place in oven and roast 1 hour, until tender. Remove from oven and cool to the touch. The skins should slip off; if not, gently peel them. Cut beets into bite-sized pieces. Note: Beets may be roasted a day ahead and kept wrapped in the refrigerator.
3. In a large serving bowl, add greens, beets, orange, mango, and almonds and toss well to combine. Set aside.
4. In a small bowl, combine lime juice, vinegar, agave, oil, mustard, cumin, and chili seasoning and whisk well to combine.
5. Pour vinaigrette over beet mixture and toss well to coat. Serve immediately.

Coconut Collards with Sweet Potatoes and Black Beans

In this recipe, the collards are bathed with a subtle sweetness from the coconut milk and a light citrus kick from the lime juice. For a spicier version, add a fresh minced jalapeño pepper or ¼ teaspoon ground cayenne while cooking.

- 1 tablespoon olive oil
- 1 medium yellow onion, peeled and chopped
- 4 cloves garlic, peeled and minced
- 2 medium carrots, peeled and sliced
- 2 medium stalks celery, trimmed and sliced
- 1 medium red bell pepper, seeded and diced
- 2 medium sweet potatoes, peeled and cubed
- 1 pound fresh collard greens, chopped
- 1 (14.5-ounce) can no-salt-added diced tomatoes, with juice
- 1 (13.5-ounce) can light coconut milk, shaken well
- 1 (15-ounce) can black beans, drained and rinsed
- ¼ cup tomato paste
- 1 tablespoon Thai red curry paste
- Juice of 2 medium limes
- 1½ teaspoons ground cumin
- 1½ teaspoons ground paprika
- ¼ teaspoon ground allspice
- ¼ teaspoon ground black pepper

Serves 8

Per Serving

Calories	178
Fat	5g
Protein	7g
Sodium	286mg
Fiber	9g
Carbohydrates	27g
Sugar	7g

1. In a large stockpot, heat oil over medium heat. Add onion, garlic, carrots, celery, bell pepper, and sweet potatoes and cook, stirring, 3 minutes, until they begin to sweat.
2. Add remaining ingredients and stir well to combine. Cover and simmer over medium heat, stirring frequently, 10 minutes.
3. Reduce heat to medium-low or low and simmer covered, stirring frequently, 5–10 minutes until sweet potatoes are fork-tender. Keep checking to make sure the mixture isn't cooking too fast or beginning to stick and burn; lower heat if necessary.
4. Remove from heat and serve immediately.

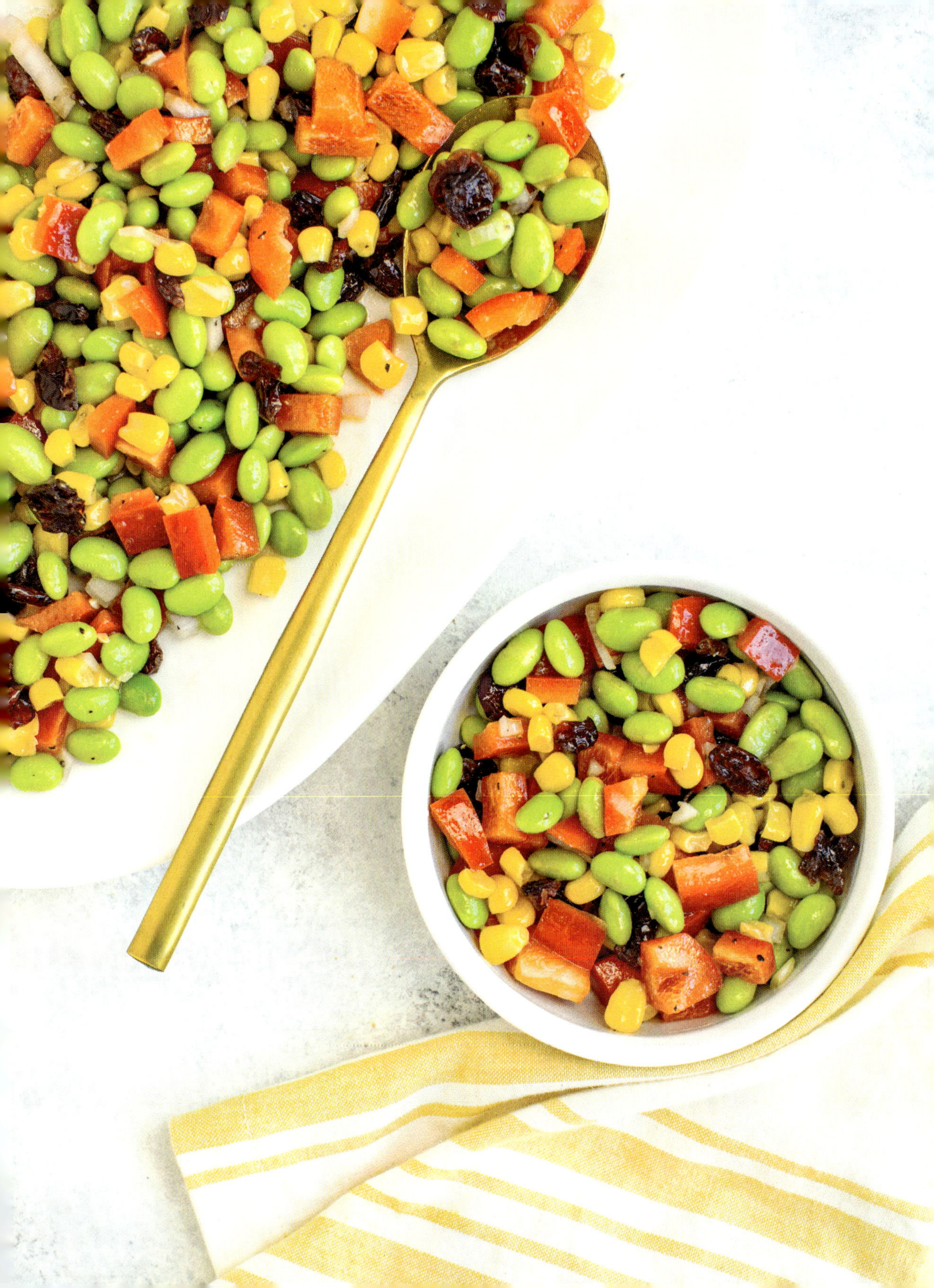

Edamame with Corn and Cranberries

A delightfully chewy, crisp, and colorful way to brighten your plate, this super-quick side is especially great for summer picnics and can be doubled or tripled to feed a crowd. Either freshly cooked corn or frozen thawed corn kernels may be used in this recipe. Dried cherries may be substituted for the cranberries if desired.

1¼ cups shelled edamame

¾ cup corn kernels

1 small red bell pepper, seeded and diced

¼ cup dried sweetened cranberries

1 medium shallot, peeled and finely diced

2 tablespoons red wine vinegar

1 tablespoon olive oil

1 teaspoon agave nectar

1 teaspoon yellow mustard

¼ teaspoon ground black pepper

Serves 4

Per Serving

Calories	155
Fat	6g
Protein	8g
Sodium	28mg
Fiber	5g
Carbohydrates	20g
Sugar	10g

1. In a medium bowl, add edamame, corn, bell pepper, cranberries, and shallot and stir to combine.
2. In a small bowl, add vinegar, oil, agave, mustard, and black pepper and whisk well.
3. Pour dressing over salad and toss well to coat. Serve immediately or cover and refrigerate until ready to serve.

Mexican Brown Rice and Beans

You can enjoy this dish as a yummy side, or as a filling for burritos, tacos, nachos, and more. Stir in sautéed bell pepper, corn, tender sweet potato, diced avocado, and more for a complete one-dish meal.

Serves 4

Per Serving

Calories	391
Fat	5g
Protein	14g
Sodium	792mg
Fiber	4g
Carbohydrates	70g
Sugar	3g

1 tablespoon olive oil

1 teaspoon ground cumin

2 teaspoons chili seasoning

1 medium red onion, peeled and diced finely

1 cup uncooked brown rice, rinsed well

2 cups vegetable broth

1 tablespoon tomato paste

2 (15-ounce) cans pinto beans, drained and rinsed

¼ teaspoon ground black pepper

¼ cup chopped fresh cilantro

1. In a medium saucepan, heat oil over medium heat. Add cumin and chili seasoning and sauté until fragrant, 30 seconds. Add onion and cook, stirring, 2 minutes, until it begins to sweat.
2. Add rice and stir well to coat. Add broth and tomato paste and combine. Bring to a boil over high heat, reduce heat to low, cover, and simmer until all the liquid is absorbed, about 40 minutes.
3. Remove pan from heat and place contents in a large serving bowl. Add beans, pepper, and cilantro to rice mixture and stir to combine. Serve immediately.

Roasted Chickpeas and Asparagus

A simple side with a ton of delicious flavor—in this dish, the chickpeas and fresh asparagus are tossed with a drizzle of sweet and salty dressing, then hot roasted. The result is a tender marriage of greens and protein you won't be able to stop devouring!

1 (15-ounce) can chickpeas, drained and rinsed

1 pound fresh asparagus, trimmed and cut into 2" pieces

2 teaspoons sesame oil

1 teaspoon low-sodium soy sauce

1 teaspoon unflavored rice wine vinegar

1 teaspoon agave nectar

¼ teaspoon ground black pepper

Serves 4

Per Serving

Calories	130
Fat	3g
Protein	6g
Sodium	171mg
Fiber	6g
Carbohydrates	19g
Sugar	5g

1. Preheat oven to 425°F. Line a baking sheet with parchment and set aside.
2. In a medium bowl, add chickpeas and asparagus. Add remaining ingredients and toss well to coat. Place mixture on baking sheet.
3. Place baking sheet on middle rack in oven and bake 20 minutes, until tender.
4. Remove from oven and serve immediately.

Refried Beans

This tasty recipe comes together so fast, you can enjoy it anytime the craving hits. Roll these beans up in tortillas with sautéed onion, peppers, and salsa or use as a spread for crackers and raw vegetables. Swap kidney or black beans for the pinto.

Serves 3

Per Serving

Calories	121
Fat	0g
Protein	7g
Sodium	221mg
Fiber	0g
Carbohydrates	22g
Sugar	0g

Pinto Bean Facts

Pinto in Spanish means "painted," which describes the speckled exterior of these tasty and nutritious beans. High in protein, folate, fiber, and minerals, pinto beans are an excellent addition to a healthy diet. Add them to chilis, soups, and salads; layer with vegetables and bake for a hot casserole; or mash to make a dip or sandwich spread.

1 (15-ounce) can pinto beans
1 teaspoon onion powder
½ teaspoon garlic powder
¼ teaspoon ground cumin
¼ teaspoon low-sodium soy sauce
¼ teaspoon ground black pepper

1. Drain beans, reserving the liquid, and rinse well.
2. In a food processor, add beans, onion powder, garlic powder, cumin, soy sauce, and pepper and pulse until smooth. Add ¼ cup of reserved bean liquid to thin if desired. Serve immediately.

Kidney Beans with Carrots, Potatoes, and Kale

This hearty, one-pot meal is filled with the earthy flavors of carrots, potatoes, and kale. The red wine adds a depth of flavor that's delicious. Serve over cooked brown rice for added heft. Spinach or collard greens may be substituted for the kale if desired.

- 1 tablespoon olive oil
- 1 medium yellow onion, peeled and diced
- 3 cloves garlic, peeled and minced
- 3 medium carrots, peeled and diced
- 2 medium stalks celery, trimmed and diced
- 2 medium potatoes, peeled and diced
- 2½ cups vegetable broth
- ½ cup red wine
- 1¼ teaspoons ground cumin
- 1 teaspoon all-purpose seasoning
- ½ teaspoon ground coriander
- ½ teaspoon dried oregano
- ¼ teaspoon dried thyme
- ¼ teaspoon ground black pepper
- 6 cups chopped fresh kale leaves
- 1 (15-ounce) can kidney beans, drained and rinsed
- 2 tablespoons lemon juice

Serves 4

Per Serving

Calories	256
Fat	4g
Protein	9g
Sodium	707mg
Fiber	10g
Carbohydrates	44g
Sugar	6g

1. In a medium stockpot, heat oil over medium heat. Add onion, garlic, carrots, and celery and cook, stirring, 5 minutes. Add potatoes, broth, wine, cumin, seasoning, coriander, oregano, thyme, and pepper and stir well to combine.
2. Bring to a boil over high heat, reduce heat to medium-low, cover pot, and simmer 15 minutes, stirring occasionally.
3. Uncover pot, add kale and beans, and stir to combine. Cover and simmer 10 minutes until kale is tender.
4. Remove from heat and stir in lemon juice. Serve immediately.

CHAPTER 9

Desserts

Sweet Corn Muffins

They're sweet, they're soft, and they're even a little crunchy on top. These muffins are an amazing dessert that makes any meal—breakfast, lunch, or dinner—better!

Serves 12

Per Serving

Calories	187
Fat	10g
Protein	2g
Sodium	136mg
Fiber	2g
Carbohydrates	24g
Sugar	8g

1 cup cornmeal

1 cup white whole-wheat flour

½ cup granulated sugar

1 tablespoon baking powder

¾ cup unsweetened almond milk

½ cup olive oil

1 teaspoon vanilla extract

1. Preheat oven to 400°F. Line a 12-cup muffin pan with paper liners and set aside.
2. In a medium bowl, add cornmeal, flour, sugar, and baking powder and whisk well to combine.
3. Add milk, oil, and vanilla and stir just until combined.
4. Divide batter evenly among muffin cups. Place pan on middle rack in oven and bake 15 minutes, until tester inserted into center of muffin comes out clean.
5. Remove from oven and place pan on a wire rack to cool. Cool 10 minutes before removing muffins from pan and placing on a wire rack to cool fully.

Maple Carrot Energy Cake

Dense, filling, and subtly sweet, this cake is packed with raisins, nuts, and carrots. It makes a great hiking snack, power breakfast, or guilt-free dessert. Bake, slice, and freeze this cake in individual zip-top sandwich bags and you have 16 wholesome brain-boosting, body-fueling bars to grab, thaw, and enjoy on the go!

- ¼ cup plus 1 teaspoon olive oil, divided
- 1 cup plus 1 tablespoon unbleached all-purpose flour, divided
- ¾ cup seedless raisins
- 1 cup pineapple juice
- 2 tablespoons ground flaxseed
- 6 tablespoons water
- 2 cups grated carrot
- ½ cup pure maple syrup
- ¼ cup unsweetened applesauce
- 1 cup white whole-wheat flour
- ¼ cup chopped walnuts
- 1 tablespoon baking powder
- 1 teaspoon ground cinnamon
- ½ teaspoon ground allspice
- ¼ teaspoon ground ginger
- ⅛ teaspoon ground cloves

1. Preheat oven to 375°F. Grease and flour an 8" square baking pan using 1 teaspoon oil and 1 tablespoon all-purpose flour and set aside.
2. In a small bowl, add raisins and pineapple juice and set aside 10 minutes to soften.
3. In a separate small bowl, add flaxseed and water and stir to combine. Set aside to thicken.
4. In a large bowl, combine raisins and pineapple juice, carrot, syrup, applesauce, and remaining ¼ cup oil.
5. In a medium bowl, add remaining 1 cup all-purpose flour, whole-wheat flour, walnuts, baking powder, cinnamon, allspice, ginger, and cloves and whisk well to combine.
6. Add flour mixture to raisin mixture, then add flaxseed mixture and stir to combine.
7. Pour batter into prepared pan. Place pan on middle rack in oven and bake until tester inserted into center comes out clean, 50–60 minutes.
8. Remove from oven and place on a wire rack to cool to touch. Cut into slices and serve.

Serves 16

Per Serving

Calories	160
Fat	5g
Protein	3g
Sodium	103mg
Fiber	2g
Carbohydrates	27g
Sugar	12g

White Whole-Wheat Flour

Hard red wheat, the type of flour used in many whole-wheat breads, is high in nutrients, but its flavor can be overpowering. White whole-wheat flour has the same health benefits as red, but with a much lighter taste and texture. It can often be used interchangeably with all-purpose flour and is a great way of boosting a recipe's fiber and nutrients without compromising taste.

Chewy Pumpkin Oatmeal Raisin Cookies

Super chewy and fabulously flavorful, these oatmeal raisin cookies are made even better by the addition of pumpkin. Soft, sweet, and amazingly delicious, you'll find yourself eating them by the handful, so watch out!

Yields 48 cookies

Per Serving (Serving size: 2 cookies)

Calories	193
Fat	7g
Protein	2g
Sodium	107mg
Fiber	2g
Carbohydrates	32g
Sugar	20g

1 cup pumpkin purée

1⅔ cups granulated sugar

2 tablespoons molasses

1½ teaspoons vanilla extract

⅔ cup olive oil

1 tablespoon ground flaxseed

2 teaspoons baking soda

1 teaspoon ground cinnamon

½ teaspoon ground nutmeg

1 cup unbleached all-purpose flour

1 cup white whole-wheat flour

1⅓ cups rolled oats

1 cup seedless raisins

1. Preheat oven to 350°F. Line two baking sheets with parchment and set aside.
2. In a large bowl, add all ingredients and stir together using a rubber spatula. Scrape the bottom and sides of the bowl to incorporate everything fully.
3. Scoop batter out by tablespoons—a small retractable ice-cream scoop works wonderfully here—and place on baking sheets.
4. Place sheets on middle rack in oven and bake 16 minutes, until golden brown. Remove from oven and transfer cookies to a wire rack to cool.
5. Repeat process with remaining batter. Store cooled cookies at room temperature in an airtight container up to 3 days.

Grilled Pineapple

Fire up the grill and get ready for a treat! Sweet, juicy pineapple gets even better with heat, transforming into a sophisticated, succulent dessert. For a spicier version, add ⅛ teaspoon ground cayenne to the marinade. This also makes a fabulous addition to fruit-based salsas; try using it in Mango Salsa (Chapter 5).

1 medium fresh pineapple
1 tablespoon agave nectar
1 tablespoon lime juice
1 tablespoon olive oil
½ teaspoon ground ginger

1. Heat the grill to medium-high.
2. Cut off the top and bottom of pineapple. Carefully remove spiky outer peel, then slice pineapple in half lengthwise. Slice each half again lengthwise to make 4 quarters. Slice down the center of each quarter to remove the hard inner core. Cut each quarter into 1" slices. Place pineapple in a large bowl.
3. In a small bowl, add remaining ingredients and whisk well to combine. Add dressing to pineapple and toss well to coat.
4. Place pineapple slices on grill and cook 5 minutes. Flip slices and grill another 5 minutes, until char marks appear on pineapple.
5. Remove from grill and serve immediately.

Serves 8

Per Serving

Calories	77
Fat	2g
Protein	1g
Sodium	1mg
Fiber	2g
Carbohydrates	16g
Sugar	12g

Cherry Blueberry Crisp

This dish is made up of ripe, luscious fruit baked beneath a sweet oatmeal crumb. Strawberries or any combination of mixed berries may be substituted for all or part of the cherries and blueberries in this recipe. If you like, top the crisp with whipped coconut cream.

Serves 8

Per Serving

Calories	235
Fat	6g
Protein	3g
Sodium	3mg
Fiber	4g
Carbohydrates	45g
Sugar	31g

3 cups sweet cherries, pitted

3 cups blueberries

1⁄3 cup granulated sugar

1 tablespoon lemon juice

1 tablespoon cornstarch

1⁄2 cup rolled oats

1⁄2 cup white whole-wheat flour

1⁄3 cup (packed) dark brown sugar

1 teaspoon ground cinnamon

1⁄4 teaspoon ground allspice

3 tablespoons olive oil

1 tablespoon vanilla extract

1. Preheat oven to 375°F. Get out a 2-quart baking pan and set aside.
2. In a large bowl, add cherries and blueberries. Add sugar, lemon juice, and cornstarch and toss well to combine. Transfer mixture to baking pan and set aside.
3. In a medium bowl, add oats, flour, brown sugar, cinnamon, and allspice and whisk well to combine. Add oil and vanilla and, using your clean hands, mix and squeeze the mixture to form a coarse crumb. Sprinkle crumb topping evenly over fruit in pan.
4. Place pan on middle rack in oven and bake 30 minutes until golden brown.
5. Remove from oven and place on a wire rack to cool. Serve warm or cool.

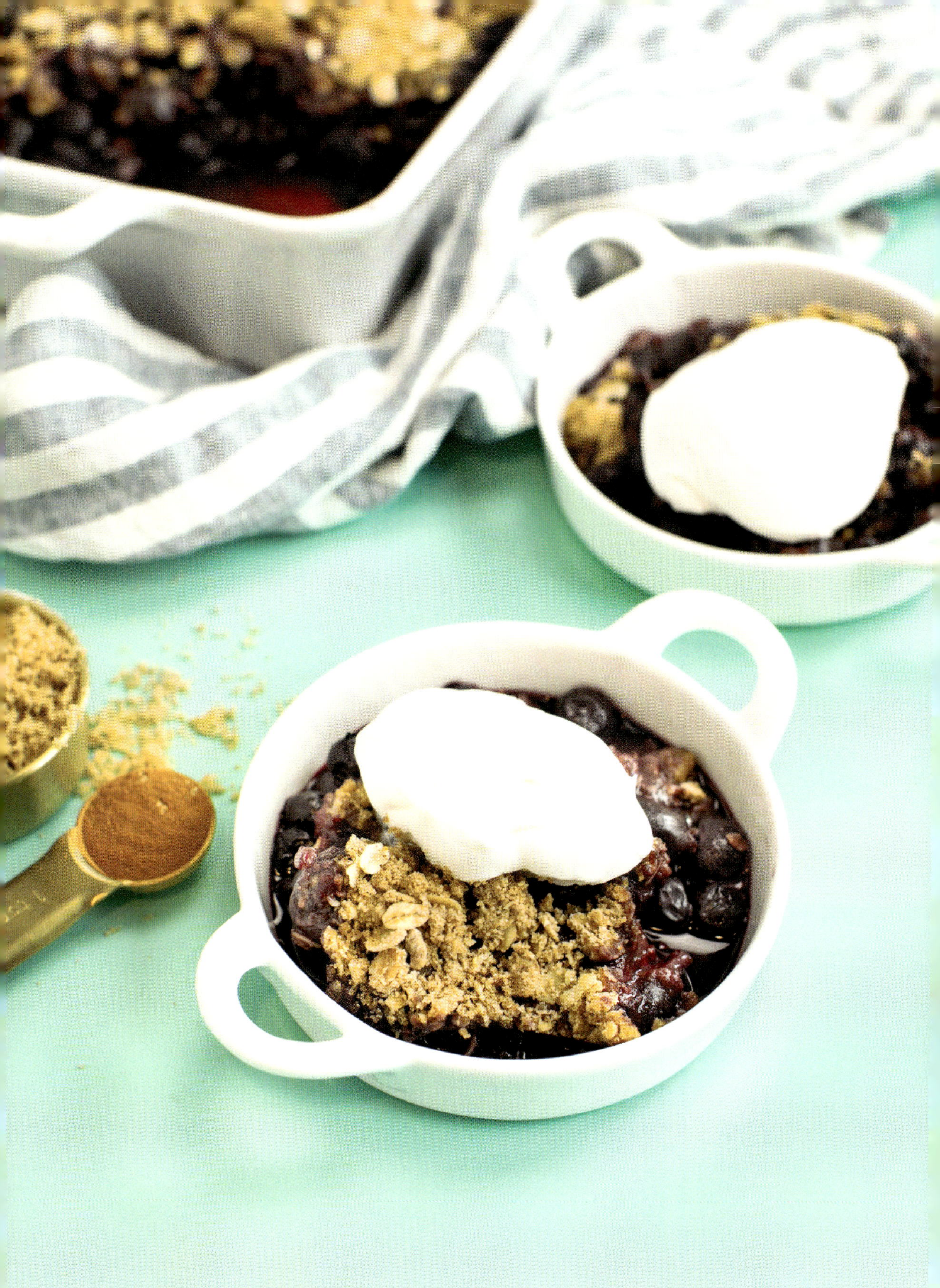

Curry Cookies

These deliciously different cookies are crisp on the outside and super soft in the middle. The combination of curry powder, peanut butter, and banana may sound strange, but it's so good! For less heat, omit the ground cayenne.

Yields 30 cookies

Per Serving (Serving size: 2 cookies)

Calories	140
Fat	6g
Protein	3g
Sodium	69mg
Fiber	2g
Carbohydrates	21g
Sugar	13g

Ice-Cream Scoops Make Perfect Cookies!

Instead of fumbling with tablespoons, scoop out cookie dough using a small retractable ice-cream scoop. Ice-cream scoops produce uniform, picture-perfect cookies and reduce the hassle and mess of working with often thick, sticky doughs and batters. Small scoops are sold in a variety of sizes at kitchenware shops and other retailers as well as online.

1 medium ripe banana, peeled and mashed
¾ cup granulated sugar
⅓ cup creamy natural peanut butter
¼ cup unsweetened almond milk
3 tablespoons olive oil
1 tablespoon molasses
1 teaspoon vanilla extract
1 cup white whole-wheat flour
2 teaspoons baking powder
1 tablespoon curry powder
½ teaspoon ground ginger
¼ teaspoon ground cardamom
⅛ teaspoon ground cayenne

1. Preheat oven to 350°F. Line two baking sheets with parchment and set aside.
2. In a medium bowl, add banana, sugar, peanut butter, milk, oil, molasses, and vanilla and stir well to combine. Add remaining ingredients and stir just until combined. The dough will be very thick and sticky.
3. Drop by tablespoonfuls onto prepared baking sheets. Place sheets on middle rack in oven and bake 12 minutes, until lightly golden.
4. Remove from oven. Transfer cookies to a wire rack to cool. Store cooled cookies in an airtight container.

Lemon Cookies

Crisp, buttery, and low in cholesterol, these deliciously simple cookies shine with bright citrus flavor. If you don't have fresh lemons, use ½ cup bottled lemon juice and ½ teaspoon lemon extract instead. Substitute lime, orange, or grapefruit juice for a twist on the same recipe.

Yields 36 cookies

Per Serving (Serving size: 1 cookie)

Calories	209
Fat	9g
Protein	2g
Sodium	27mg
Fiber	1g
Carbohydrates	30g
Sugar	17g

1½ cups unbleached all-purpose flour

1 cup white whole-wheat flour

1½ cups granulated sugar

1 tablespoon baking powder

¾ cup olive oil

Grated zest and juice of 2 large lemons

1 tablespoon vanilla extract

1. Preheat oven to 350°F. Take out two baking sheets and set aside.
2. In a medium bowl, add flours, sugar, and baking powder and whisk well to combine. Add remaining ingredients and stir to form a stiff dough.
3. Drop by rounded tablespoons onto the ungreased baking sheets. Place sheets on middle rack in oven and bake 10 minutes, until cookies are pale and have spread out.
4. Remove from oven, cool on baking sheets a few minutes, then transfer to a wire rack to cool fully.
5. Serve cooled cookies or store in an airtight container up to 3 days.

Chocolate Gingerbread

This amazingly moist, cocoa-spiked gingerbread is simply delicious. If caffeine is an issue for you, use an equal amount of decaffeinated coffee for the traditional brew. If you don't have crystallized ginger on hand, substitute chocolate chips, raisins, or chopped dried fruit instead.

Serves 16

Per Serving

Calories	161
Fat	7g
Protein	2g
Sodium	65mg
Fiber	1g
Carbohydrates	24g
Sugar	15g

½ cup plus 1 teaspoon olive oil, divided
⅓ cup unsweetened cocoa powder
⅔ cup unbleached all-purpose flour
⅔ cup white whole-wheat flour
1 cup (packed) dark brown sugar
2 teaspoons baking powder
2½ teaspoons ground ginger
1 teaspoon ground cinnamon
1 cup brewed coffee, cooled to room temperature
¼ cup chopped crystallized ginger
2 tablespoons apple cider vinegar

1. Preheat oven to 375°F. Lightly oil an 8" square baking pan with 1 teaspoon olive oil and dust with a tiny amount of flour or cocoa powder. Set aside.
2. In a medium bowl, add cocoa powder, flours, sugar, baking powder, ground ginger, and cinnamon and whisk well to combine. Add coffee, remaining ½ cup oil, crystallized ginger, and vinegar and stir just until combined.
3. Pour batter into prepared pan. Place pan on middle rack in oven and bake 30 minutes, until tester inserted into center comes out clean.
4. Remove pan from oven and place on a wire rack to cool. Slice into squares and serve.

Fresh Pear Cake with Cardamom and Pecans

Light, airy, and fragrant, this moist and flavorful cake is sure to be one of your favorites. Apples may be substituted for a portion of the pears; try baking different combinations, with different types of pears and apples, and decide which you like best.

- ½ cup plus 1 teaspoon olive oil, divided
- 1 cup plus 1 tablespoon unbleached all-purpose flour, divided
- 3 medium pears, peeled, cored, and chopped
- ⅔ cup granulated sugar
- 2 tablespoons lemon juice
- 1 tablespoon ground flaxseed
- 3 tablespoons water
- ¼ cup white whole-wheat flour
- 1 tablespoon baking powder
- ½ teaspoon ground cardamom
- ¼ cup chopped pecans
- 1½ teaspoons almond extract
- 1½ teaspoons vanilla extract

Serves 16

Per Serving

Calories	165
Fat	8g
Protein	1g
Sodium	92mg
Fiber	2g
Carbohydrates	22g
Sugar	12g

1. Preheat oven to 375°F. Grease and flour an 8" square baking pan with 1 teaspoon olive oil and 1 tablespoon all-purpose flour and set aside.
2. In a medium bowl, add pears, sugar, and lemon juice and stir to combine. Set aside.
3. In a small bowl, add flaxseed and water and stir to combine. Set aside to thicken.
4. In a separate medium bowl, add remaining 1 cup all-purpose flour, whole-wheat flour, baking powder, cardamom, and pecans and whisk well to combine.
5. To pear mixture, add flaxseed mixture, remaining ½ cup oil, and almond and vanilla extracts and stir well. Add in flour mixture and stir until combined. The batter will be very thick and sticky.
6. Pour batter into prepared pan and spread to even it. Place pan on middle rack in oven and bake 35 minutes, until golden brown.
7. Remove pan from oven and place on a wire rack to cool. Slice into squares and serve.

Pear Facts

Eaten raw, cooked, and dried, pears are also prized for their delicious juice, which can be fermented into an alcoholic cider. When enjoying fresh pears, wash and consume without peeling; the skin contains important phytonutrients and fiber. Unripe pears should be stored at room temperature; once ripe, they should be refrigerated. Test for ripeness by pressing gently around the stem and neck; ripe, juicy pears will yield to gentle pressure.

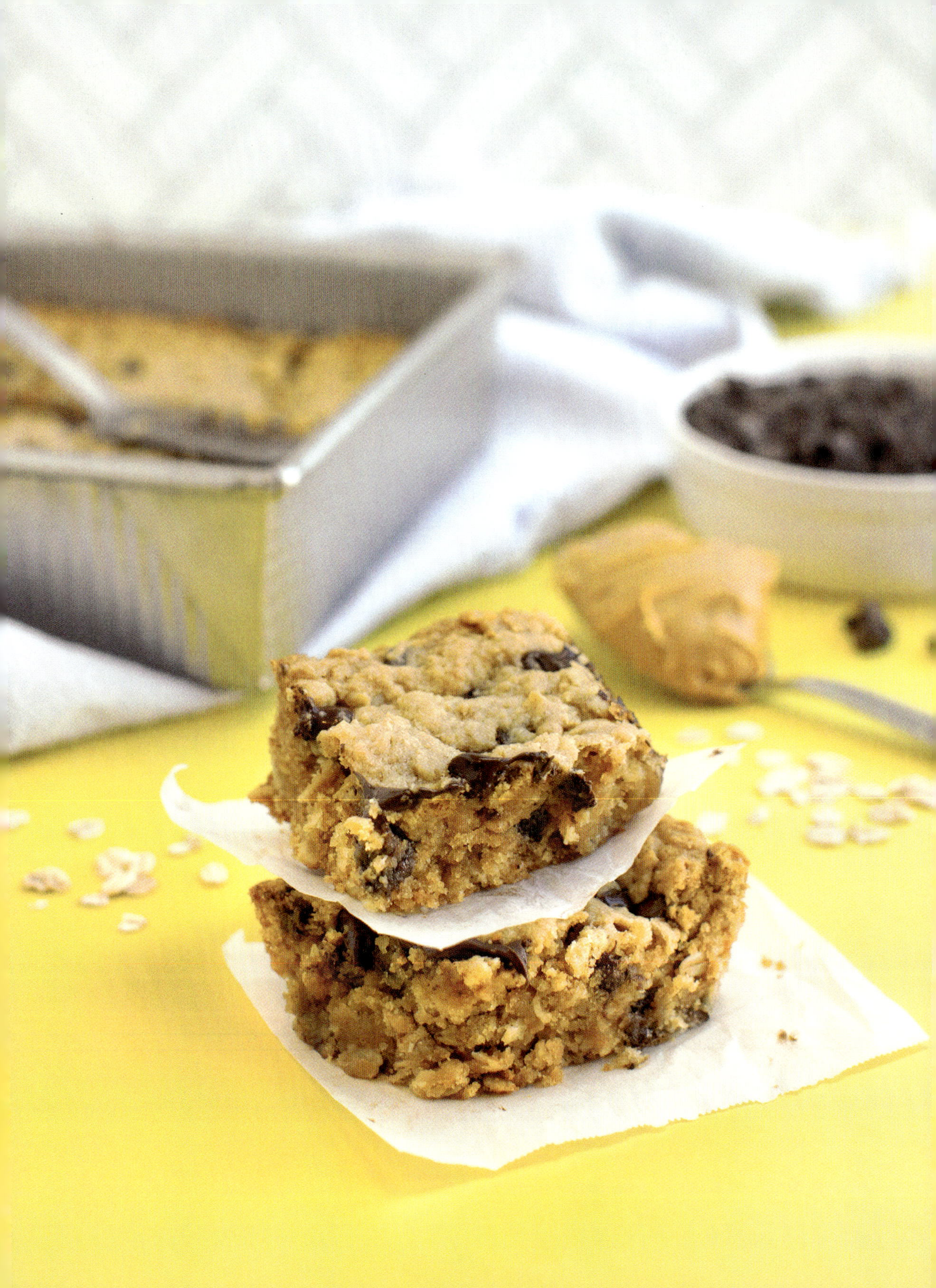

Peanut Butter Chocolate Chip Blondies

Peanut butter and chocolate make a mouthwatering combination in these chewy cookie bars. For extra crunch, sprinkle a tablespoon of chopped unsalted peanuts on top of the batter before baking. For brownie bars, reduce the all-purpose flour to ¼ cup and add ¼ cup unsweetened cocoa powder.

6 tablespoons plus 1 teaspoon olive oil, divided
½ cup unbleached all-purpose flour
½ cup white whole-wheat flour
1 cup quick oats
½ cup (packed) dark brown sugar
½ cup granulated sugar
2 teaspoons baking powder
½ cup creamy natural peanut butter
½ cup vanilla almond milk
1 tablespoon vanilla extract
½ cup semisweet chocolate chips

1. Preheat oven to 350°F. Lightly oil an 8" square baking pan with 1 teaspoon oil and set aside.
2. In a medium bowl, add flours, oats, sugars, and baking powder and whisk well to combine. Add remaining 6 tablespoons oil, peanut butter, milk, vanilla, and chocolate chips and stir well to combine. Press dough into prepared pan.
3. Place pan on middle rack in oven and bake 35 minutes, until golden brown.
4. Remove from oven and place on a wire rack to cool fully. Cut into bars and serve.

Serves 16

Per Serving

Calories	254
Fat	13g
Protein	4g
Sodium	79mg
Fiber	2g
Carbohydrates	32g
Sugar	20g

Cookie Bar Baking Tip

When baking cookie bars, allow them to fully cool in the pan before slicing and removing. This keeps the edges intact and helps ensure your cookie bars look picture-perfect. To get evenly sized bars, slice halfway through the pan, then divide each half in half and slice again.

Whole-Grain Strawberry Bread

A fabulous, fruit-filled quick bread that is summer fresh! It's moist with juicy bits of strawberry and has an irresistible cinnamon scent. Spread with peanut butter for a delicious PB&J-inspired sandwich—no jelly needed.

Serves 16

Per Serving

Calories	173
Fat	10g
Protein	2g
Sodium	87mg
Fiber	1g
Carbohydrates	20g
Sugar	10g

Cut the Fat!

When looking to minimize oil in baked goods, try substituting unsweetened applesauce, mashed banana, or puréed prunes for all or part of the fat. When sautéing, coat the bottom of pans with water or broth. Little steps like these add up and will keep you healthier.

2⁄3 cup plus 1 teaspoon olive oil, divided

1 cup unbleached all-purpose flour

1⁄2 cup white whole-wheat flour

1 1⁄4 cups mashed fresh strawberries

3⁄4 cup granulated sugar

2 large eggs, beaten

2 teaspoons ground cinnamon

1 teaspoon baking soda

1. Preheat oven to 350°F. Grease an 8" × 3" loaf pan with 1 teaspoon oil and set aside.
2. In a large bowl, add all ingredients and stir just until combined. Pour batter into the prepared pan.
3. Place pan on middle rack in oven and bake 1 hour, until tester inserted into center comes out clean.
4. Remove from oven and place pan on a wire rack to cool. Serve warm or at room temperature.

Oven-Baked Apple Pancake

Moist, airy, and delicious, this homey dessert will impress with its taste and simplicity. The oven does all the work; just whisk together the ingredients, pour, and bake. For variety, substitute diced pears, plums, or peaches for the apple, or add chopped nuts or dried fruit to the batter. Serve for breakfast or brunch too!

1 teaspoon olive oil

2 cups peeled, cored, and diced apple

1 tablespoon vanilla extract

1 tablespoon baking powder

½ cup unbleached all-purpose flour

½ cup white whole-wheat flour

⅓ cup unsweetened applesauce

⅓ cup plus ¼ cup (for drizzling) pure maple syrup, divided

¾ cup unsweetened almond milk

1 tablespoon granulated sugar

½ teaspoon ground cinnamon

Serves 8

Per Serving

Calories	149
Fat	1g
Protein	2g
Sodium	202mg
Fiber	2g
Carbohydrates	34g
Sugar	19g

1. Preheat oven to 400°F. Lightly coat a large ovenproof skillet with oil and set aside.
2. In a medium bowl, add apple, vanilla, baking powder, flours, applesauce, ⅓ cup syrup, and milk and whisk well to combine. Pour batter into the prepared skillet and smooth top to even it.
3. In a small bowl, combine sugar and cinnamon and sprinkle evenly over batter.
4. Place skillet on middle rack in oven and bake 25 minutes, until golden brown.
5. Remove skillet from oven. Use a rubber spatula and carefully loosen pancake from pan. Slice like a pizza into 8 pieces, drizzle with remaining ¼ cup syrup, and serve immediately.

Jam-Filled Cupcakes

These light and fluffy cupcakes make eating on the MIND diet fun. The jam keeps them moist, so there's no need to frost. Add ½ teaspoon lemon, orange, or maple extract instead of the almond, and play around with different jams to find your favorite flavor combinations.

Serves 12

Per Serving

Calories	163
Fat	6g
Protein	2g
Sodium	134mg
Fiber	1g
Carbohydrates	25g
Sugar	12g

Desserts and the MIND Diet

People often equate dieting with deprivation, but sweets can be part of a healthy lifestyle when chosen wisely and consumed in moderation. If you're someone with an above-average sweet tooth, try to channel cravings into the healthy realm of fruit. Dried fruit, applesauce, and juice-sweetened fruit cups also make great guilt-free snacks.

- ⅔ cup unsweetened almond milk
- ½ teaspoon apple cider vinegar
- ⅔ cup agave nectar
- ⅓ cup olive oil
- 1½ teaspoons vanilla extract
- ½ teaspoon almond extract
- 1 cup unbleached all-purpose flour
- ⅓ cup white whole-wheat flour
- 1 tablespoon baking powder
- ¼ cup strawberry jam, at room temperature

1. Preheat oven to 325°F. Line a 12-cup muffin pan with paper liners and set aside.
2. In a medium bowl, add milk and vinegar. Stir well and set aside 5 minutes to curdle.
3. Add agave, oil, and vanilla and almond extracts to milk-vinegar mixture and stir well to combine. Add flours and baking powder and whisk until smooth.
4. Fill each muffin cup with 2 tablespoons batter, top with 1 teaspoon jam, then cover with another 2 tablespoons batter. Try to get the jam in the center of the muffin cup so it's not creeping out the sides and be sure to cover the jam completely.
5. Place pan on middle rack in oven and bake 22 minutes, until golden brown.
6. Remove pan from oven and place on a wire rack to cool before serving. Cool 10 minutes, then carefully remove cupcakes from pan and place on wire rack to cool fully.

Chocolate-Covered Strawberries

These elegant treats are so easy to make at home. For an extra-fancy treat, sprinkle the freshly dipped strawberries with colored sugar or sprinkles, or drizzle with melted white chocolate. If you don't have a microwave, place the chocolate chips and oil into a double boiler and gently melt over low heat, stirring constantly.

3⁄4 cup semisweet chocolate chips

1 tablespoon olive oil

16 fresh strawberries, washed and dried completely

1. Line a baking sheet or tray with waxed paper and set it aside.
2. In a small microwave-safe bowl or mug, add chocolate chips and oil. Microwave 1 minute on high, then remove and stir constantly until chocolate is fully melted and smooth.
3. Dip each strawberry into chocolate, then place on the waxed paper. Let strawberries rest at least 10 minutes to harden. Strawberries may be refrigerated and are best consumed within a day.

Serves 8

Per Serving

Calories	104
Fat	7g
Protein	1g
Sodium	2mg
Fiber	1g
Carbohydrates	13g
Sugar	10g

Peppermint Watermelon Granita

This refreshing dessert is the perfect end to a summer meal. To serve, scoop into glasses or bowls and garnish with fresh mint leaves and extra cubed watermelon. Play around with this base recipe using different flavors of tea or juice and fruit.

Serves 6

Per Serving

Calories	30
Fat	0g
Protein	0g
Sodium	1mg
Fiber	0g
Carbohydrates	8g
Sugar	6g

3 peppermint tea bags
3 cups boiling water
3 cups cubed fresh watermelon
1 tablespoon agave nectar

1. Place tea bags in a heatproof pitcher or teapot. Add boiling water and steep 5 minutes.
2. Place watermelon in a food processor and purée.
3. Remove tea bags and pour liquid into a 9" × 13" freezer-safe pan.
4. Add watermelon and agave and stir to combine. Cover tightly with plastic wrap and place in freezer.
5. Freeze 2–3 hours, until semi-solid. Remove from freezer and scrape mixture into glasses or bowls. Serve immediately.

Watermelon Facts

Watermelon is low in fat, a good source of fiber, and as its name suggests, one of the juiciest fruits around. Watermelon contains high levels of vitamins A and C as well as lycopene, a cancer-fighting antioxidant. To select a perfectly ripe watermelon, hold it close to your body and thump firmly. If it sounds and feels hollow, it's a keeper. Put back any watermelons without reverb; they tend to be mealy.

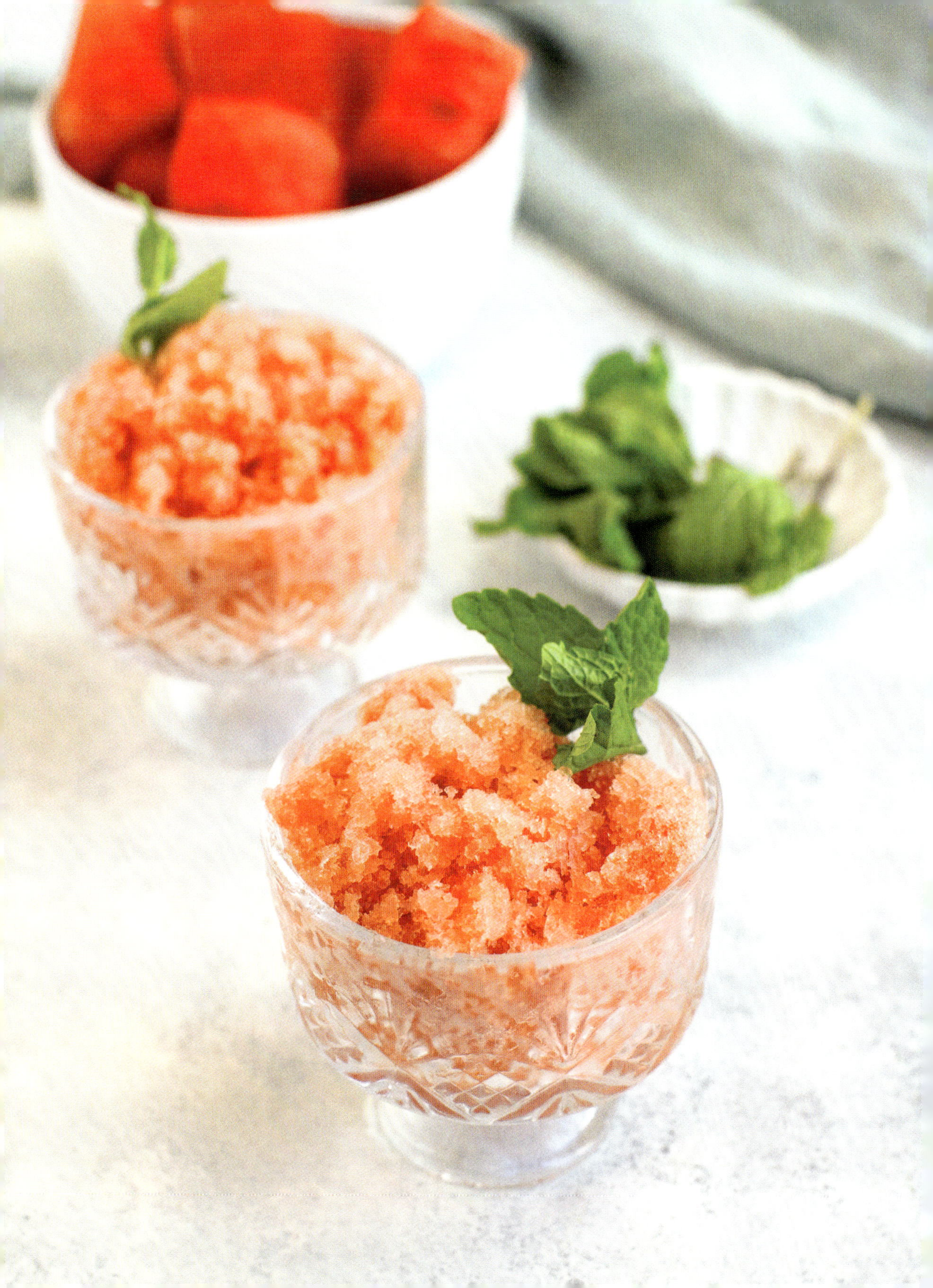

Homemade Banana Ice Cream

This dessert contains only one ingredient: bananas! Yet when frozen and puréed, the crystallized fruit so perfectly mimics the look, taste, and texture of soft-serve ice cream that it's almost magic. And for an even tastier treat, see the sidebar to learn how to top your ice cream with your very own homemade chocolate shell!

Serves 4

Per Serving

Calories	105
Fat	0g
Protein	1g
Sodium	1mg
Fiber	3g
Carbohydrates	27g
Sugar	14g

4 medium ripe bananas

1. Peel bananas, slice into chunks, place in a large zip-top plastic bag, and place in freezer. Freeze until solid.
2. Remove bananas from freezer. Place chunks in a food processor and pulse until smooth.
3. Scoop mixture out and serve immediately.

Homemade Chocolate Shell

If you love the taste and texture of that magical chocolate shell sold in stores and ice-cream parlors, here's how to make your own at home. Simply measure ½ cup semisweet chocolate chips into a microwave-safe bowl or mug, add 1 teaspoon olive oil, and microwave for 1 minute on high. Stir until smooth and drizzle over your favorite frozen dessert. It hardens almost instantly!

Foolproof Brownies

This dish gives you rich, dense, and supremely chocolatey brownies that can be enjoyed as an occasional treat. Dutch-processed cocoa produces a much deeper, more complex flavor, but standard cocoa works just fine too. Add ¼ cup chopped nuts to the batter if desired.

⅓ cup plus 1 teaspoon olive oil, divided

¾ cup plus 1 tablespoon unbleached all-purpose flour, divided

3 large eggs

1½ cups granulated sugar

1 teaspoon vanilla extract

1 cup unsweetened cocoa powder

½ cup unsalted butter, melted

1 cup semisweet chocolate chips

1. Preheat oven to 350°F. Grease and flour the bottom and sides of a 9" × 13" baking pan with 1 teaspoon oil and 1 tablespoon flour and set aside.
2. In a medium bowl, beat together eggs, sugar, and vanilla. Add cocoa, butter, and remaining ⅓ cup oil and mix well. Stir in remaining ¾ cup flour, then add chocolate chips. Scrape the bottom of the bowl to make sure everything is well incorporated.
3. Spread the thick batter into the prepared pan and smooth the top to even it out. Place on middle rack in oven and bake exactly 30 minutes (do not bake any longer!). Even if the brownies appear a little loose in the center, they will firm up fully after cooling.
4. Remove pan from oven and place on a wire rack to cool completely. Cut into slices and serve only after brownies have completely cooled.

Yields 24 brownies

Per Serving (Serving size: 1 brownie)

Calories	174
Fat	10g
Protein	2g
Sodium	11mg
Fiber	2g
Carbohydrates	22g
Sugar	17g

What Is Cocoa Powder?

Cocoa powder comes from the leftover solids that remain after cocoa butter is extracted from cacao beans. These crumbly residual bits are ground into a fine powder, making cocoa. Standard cocoa powder is slightly acidic, with a pH between 5 and 6. Dutch-processed cocoa is washed with a solution of potassium carbonate that changes its acidity, leaving it with a neutral pH of 7 or slightly alkaline pH of 8. The process changes the cocoa, giving it a darker brown color and more intense chocolate flavor.

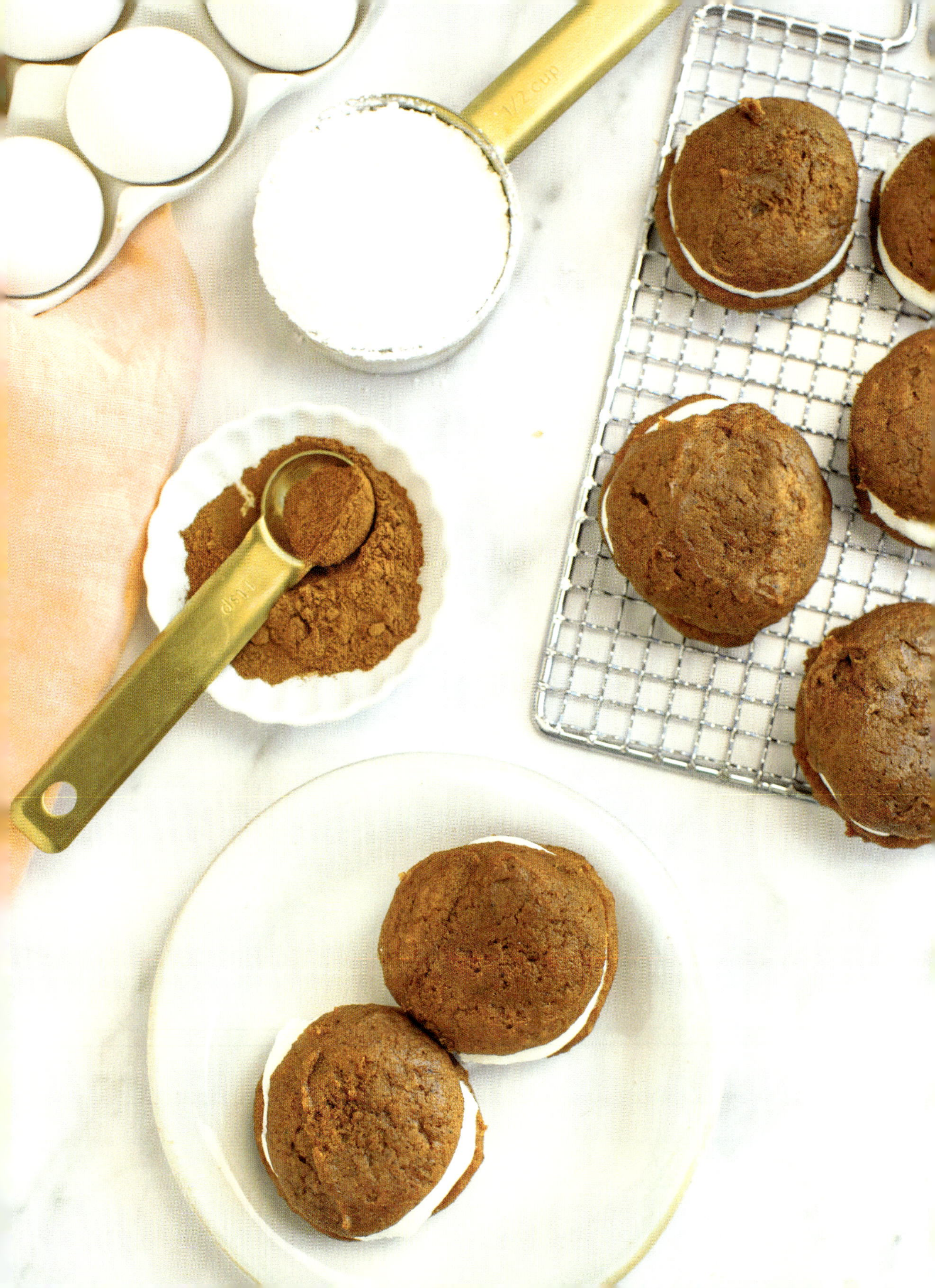
1/2 cup
1 tsp

Pumpkin Whoopie Pies

Spicy, moist, and irresistible, these whoopie pies are packed with vitamin-rich pumpkin and a sweet cream cheese filling. Due to the sugar in this recipe, these whoopies are more of a special treat than an everyday occurrence, but they are delicious so enjoy them when you can.

- 2½ cups unbleached all-purpose flour
- ½ cup white whole-wheat flour
- 2 teaspoons baking powder
- 1 teaspoon baking soda
- 2 tablespoons ground cinnamon
- 1 tablespoon ground ginger
- 1 tablespoon ground cloves
- 2 cups (packed) dark brown sugar
- 1 cup olive oil
- 3 cups pumpkin purée, chilled
- 2 large eggs
- 2 teaspoons vanilla extract, divided
- 3 cups confectioners' sugar
- 4 tablespoons unsalted butter, softened
- 2 ounces cream cheese, softened
- ¼ cup low-fat milk

Yields 12 whoopie pies

Per Serving (Serving size: 1 whoopie pie)

Calories	606
Fat	24g
Protein	6g
Sodium	233mg
Fiber	4g
Carbohydrates	92g
Sugar	63g

1. Preheat oven to 350°F. Line two baking sheets with parchment and set aside.
2. In a large bowl, whisk together flours, baking powder, baking soda, cinnamon, ginger, and cloves. Set aside.
3. In another large bowl, mix together brown sugar and oil. Add pumpkin and stir until combined. Add eggs and 1 teaspoon vanilla and mix until well combined. Gradually add flour mixture and stir until fully incorporated.
4. Use a small retractable ice-cream scoop and drop heaping tablespoons of dough onto the prepared baking sheets about 1" apart. Transfer to oven and bake on middle rack 15 minutes, until set. Remove from oven and let cool completely on baking sheet, roughly 30 minutes.
5. To make the filling, sift confectioners' sugar into a small bowl. Add butter and cream cheese and beat until smooth. Add milk and remaining 1 teaspoon vanilla and beat until fluffy.
6. When cookies have cooled completely, pipe or spread a large dollop of filling on the flat side of one of the cookies. Sandwich with another cookie and press down slightly so that the filling spreads to the edges. Transfer to a plate or cover with plastic wrap. Repeat with remaining cookies and filling.
7. Serve immediately or cover cookies with plastic wrap and refrigerate up to 3 days.

Mango Crumble

Sink your teeth into tender chunks of mango and a cinnamon-scented crust with this MIND diet favorite! For a juicier filling, omit the cornstarch. Can't find mangoes? Substitute 4 cups fresh or canned pineapple chunks, peaches, blueberries, strawberries, or another favorite fruit instead.

Serves 8

Per Serving

Calories	172
Fat	1g
Protein	3g
Sodium	1mg
Fiber	3g
Carbohydrates	41g
Sugar	27g

2 large mangoes, peeled, cored, and cut into 1" chunks

2 tablespoons dark brown sugar

1 tablespoon cornstarch

1½ teaspoons minced fresh ginger

½ cup unbleached all-purpose flour

½ cup white whole-wheat flour

½ cup granulated sugar

1 teaspoon ground cinnamon

½ teaspoon ground ginger

3 tablespoons olive oil

1. Preheat oven to 375°F. Take out an 8" square baking pan and set aside.
2. In a medium bowl, add mangoes, brown sugar, cornstarch, and fresh ginger and toss well to coat. Turn mixture out into the baking pan and spread it out evenly.
3. In another medium bowl, whisk together flours, granulated sugar, cinnamon, and ground ginger. Add oil and squeeze the mixture with your hands to form a coarse sand-like crumb. Sprinkle mixture evenly over fruit.
4. Place pan on middle rack in oven and bake 25 minutes until fruit is tender.
5. Remove from oven and place on a wire rack to cool. Serve warm or cool.

Chocolate-Drizzled Almond Biscotti

These delicious Italian cookies have a double dose of almond, with extract in the batter and slivered nuts on top. If you own an electric mixer, use it when making this batter; it'll save your arm a good workout.

½ cup plus 2 teaspoons olive oil, divided

1 cup granulated sugar

1 tablespoon vanilla extract

1½ teaspoons almond extract

3 large eggs

1 tablespoon baking powder

3½ cups unbleached all-purpose flour

½ cup semisweet chocolate chips

¼ cup chopped or slivered almonds

Yields 30 biscotti

Per Serving (Serving size: 1 biscotti)

Calories	140
Fat	5g
Protein	2g
Sodium	56mg
Fiber	1g
Carbohydrates	20g
Sugar	8g

1. Preheat oven to 375°F. Lightly grease two baking sheets with 1 teaspoon olive oil and set aside.
2. In a large bowl, beat sugar with ½ cup oil, vanilla, and almond extract. Add eggs one at a time and beat well after each addition. Stir in baking powder. Gradually add in flour and mix well, scraping the sides of the bowl to incorporate.
3. Lightly flour your hands, then divide the dough into 2 equal parts. The dough may be sticky—this is normal. Just lightly reflour your hands as necessary.
4. Roll each dough part into a roughly 8"-long cylinder. Place cylinders onto individual baking sheets, then lightly press each cylinder down to flatten to about 1½" thickness.
5. Place baking sheets on middle rack in oven and bake 25 minutes.
6. Remove sheets from oven, let rest 1 minute, then carefully slice the baked loaves with a serrated knife into 1" slices.
7. Gently place the cookies cut-side down onto the baking sheets. Place sheets on middle rack in oven and bake 5 minutes. Gently flip cookies over and bake 3 minutes until lightly toasted. Remove from oven and carefully transfer cookies to a wire rack.
8. Place chocolate chips and the remaining 1 teaspoon oil in a microwave-safe bowl or mug. Microwave 40 seconds on high. Remove from microwave and stir until smooth. Heat another 10 seconds if chips have not melted fully.
9. Drizzle chocolate over cookies and immediately sprinkle with almonds.
10. Let cookies rest until chocolate has completely hardened, then store in an airtight container up to 5 days. To speed up hardening of chocolate, place cookies in the refrigerator or freezer 10 minutes.

CHAPTER 10

Drinks

Vitamin C Juice

Feeling run-down and need a burst of energy stat? Skip the supplement pills and powders and get a natural boost from this heavenly peach-colored concoction. Each 6.5-ounce serving contains more than 160 percent of the daily recommended intake of vitamin C, almost half the daily value of vitamin A, and more.

Serves 4

Per Serving (Serving size: 6.5 ounces)

Calories	137
Fat	1g
Protein	3g
Sodium	13mg
Fiber	0g
Carbohydrates	35g
Sugar	32g

2 cups cubed fresh pineapple

1 cup fresh strawberries, trimmed

1 medium orange, peeled

1 medium mango, peeled and cored

1 medium lemon, peeled

½ medium cantaloupe, peeled and seeded

½ medium grapefruit, peeled

1. In a juicer, process ingredients according to juicer instructions.
2. Stir well to combine. Serve immediately or store in an airtight container, refrigerate, and drink within a day. Shake or stir well before using.

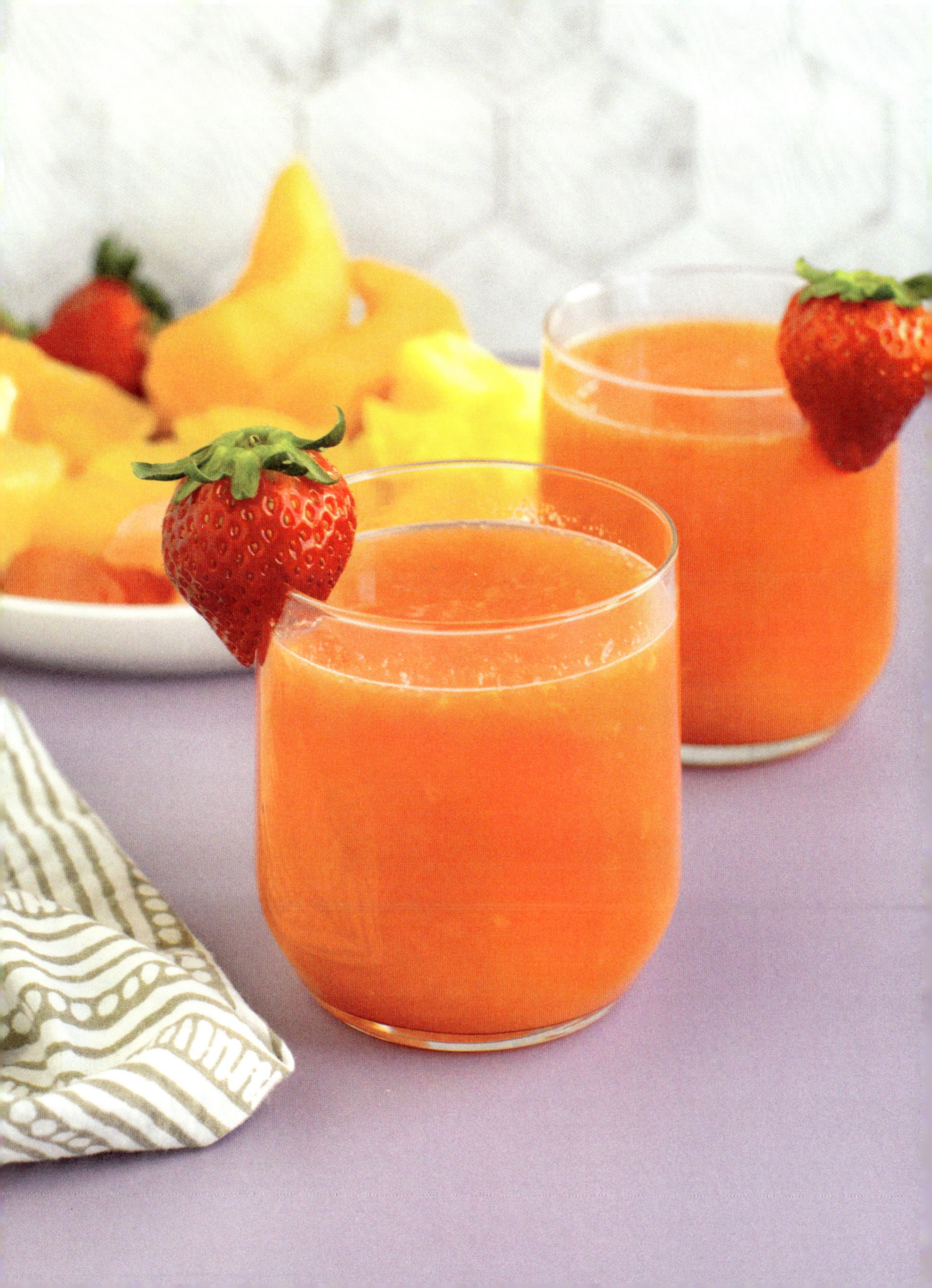

Vitamin A Juice

This green juice is delicious, with its delightful, sweet taste and garden-fresh scent. Packed with vitamin A, each 6-ounce serving contains almost five times the daily recommended value! This juice is also a great source of vitamin C and manganese.

Serves 3

Per Serving (Serving size: 6 ounces)

Calories	153
Fat	1g
Protein	4g
Sodium	77mg
Fiber	0g
Carbohydrates	37g
Sugar	35g

Vitamin A Facts

Vitamin A is a type of antioxidant found in many foods; the most prevalent form in fruits and vegetables is beta-carotene. Vitamin A is essential for good vision, especially at night, as it aids in the formation of pigments that control how well your eyes adjust in the dark. Vitamin A is also critical to the immune system, as it controls the production of white blood cells that fight infection in the body.

3 medium carrots

½ medium cantaloupe, peeled and seeded

1 medium mango, peeled and cored

1 medium orange, peeled

2 cups (packed) fresh baby spinach

2 cups (packed) chopped fresh kale leaves

1 cup cubed fresh pineapple

1. In a juicer, process ingredients according to juicer instructions.
2. Stir well to combine. Serve immediately or store in an airtight container, refrigerate, and drink within a day. Shake or stir well before using.

Homemade Vegetable Juice

This additive-free juice has an appealing orange-red color and light refreshing taste. Delicious on its own, it can also be spiked (think Bloody Mary) or seasoned to taste in a multitude of ways. Use it in lieu of or in combination with broth in any recipe.

3 medium tomatoes

2 medium carrots

2 medium stalks celery, trimmed

1 medium red bell pepper, seeded

1 medium cucumber, peeled

2 cups (packed) fresh baby spinach

½ medium yellow onion, peeled

1 medium lemon, peeled

3 cloves garlic, peeled

¼ cup fresh cilantro

1. In a juicer, process ingredients according to juicer instructions.
2. Stir well to combine. Serve immediately or store in an airtight container, refrigerate, and drink within a day. Shake or stir well before using.

Serves 5

Per Serving (Serving size: 6 ounces)

Calories	40
Fat	0g
Protein	2g
Sodium	45mg
Fiber	0g
Carbohydrates	9g
Sugar	6g

Make It Your Own!

Fresh juices and smoothies can be altered easily to correspond with the seasons and personal taste. When trying out completely new flavoring, start small and work your way up, ⅛ teaspoon at a time, until you reach a level you enjoy. For example, try flavoring this vegetable juice with spices such as ground cumin, coriander, cayenne, or black pepper, and a splash of hot sauce or low-sodium soy sauce.

PB&J Smoothie

This rich, deeply purple-hued smoothie is reminiscent of a peanut butter and jelly sandwich. It's jam-packed with brain-boosting vitamins and nutrients. Regular Concord grape juice may be substituted for all or part of the white grape juice if desired. For a thicker, more shake-like smoothie, add a peeled, frozen banana to the mix.

Serves 4

Per Serving (Serving size: 6 ounces)

Calories	165
Fat	7g
Protein	3g
Sodium	17mg
Fiber	3g
Carbohydrates	26g
Sugar	21g

1 cup frozen blueberries

½ medium ripe avocado, peeled and pitted

2 tablespoons creamy natural peanut butter

1 cup (packed) fresh baby spinach

1 cup 100% pomegranate juice

1 cup 100% white grape juice

In a food processor, add blueberries, avocado, peanut butter, and spinach and pulse to combine. Add fruit juices and pulse until smooth. Serve immediately.

Creamy "Milk" Shake

Ripe banana and avocado stand in for dairy in this super-thick and creamy guilt-free green milkshake. It's a delicious treat to enjoy anytime. Filling yet refreshing, this shake is packed with nutrients, including vitamins A, B_6, C, and E, plus folate, copper, calcium, iron, and more.

Serves 3

Per Serving (Serving size: 8 ounces)

Calories	205
Fat	3g
Protein	2g
Sodium	20mg
Fiber	4g
Carbohydrates	46g
Sugar	34g

2 medium ripe bananas, peeled

½ medium ripe avocado, peeled and pitted

1 cup (packed) fresh baby spinach

2 cups 100% white grape juice

Juice of 1 medium lemon

In a food processor, add bananas, avocado, and spinach and pulse to combine. Add fruit juices and pulse until smooth. Serve immediately.

Green Zinger Smoothie

This delicious, light, and refreshing juice is chock-full of the good stuff: two times the daily recommended value of vitamin A, and almost a full day's vitamin C, plus vitamins B_6 and E, calcium, copper, folate, iron, magnesium, manganese, and more.

2 cups (packed) fresh baby spinach

2 cups (packed) chopped fresh kale leaves

1 medium cucumber, peeled

2 medium stalks celery, trimmed

3 medium apples, cored

1 medium lime, peeled

½ medium ruby red grapefruit, peeled

¼ cup fresh cilantro

1 (1½") piece fresh ginger

Serves 4

Per Serving (Serving size: 7 ounces)

Calories	97
Fat	0g
Protein	2g
Sodium	32mg
Fiber	4g
Carbohydrates	25g
Sugar	16g

1. In a juicer, process ingredients according to juicer instructions.
2. Stir well to combine. Serve immediately or store in an airtight container, refrigerate, and drink within a day. Shake or stir well before using.

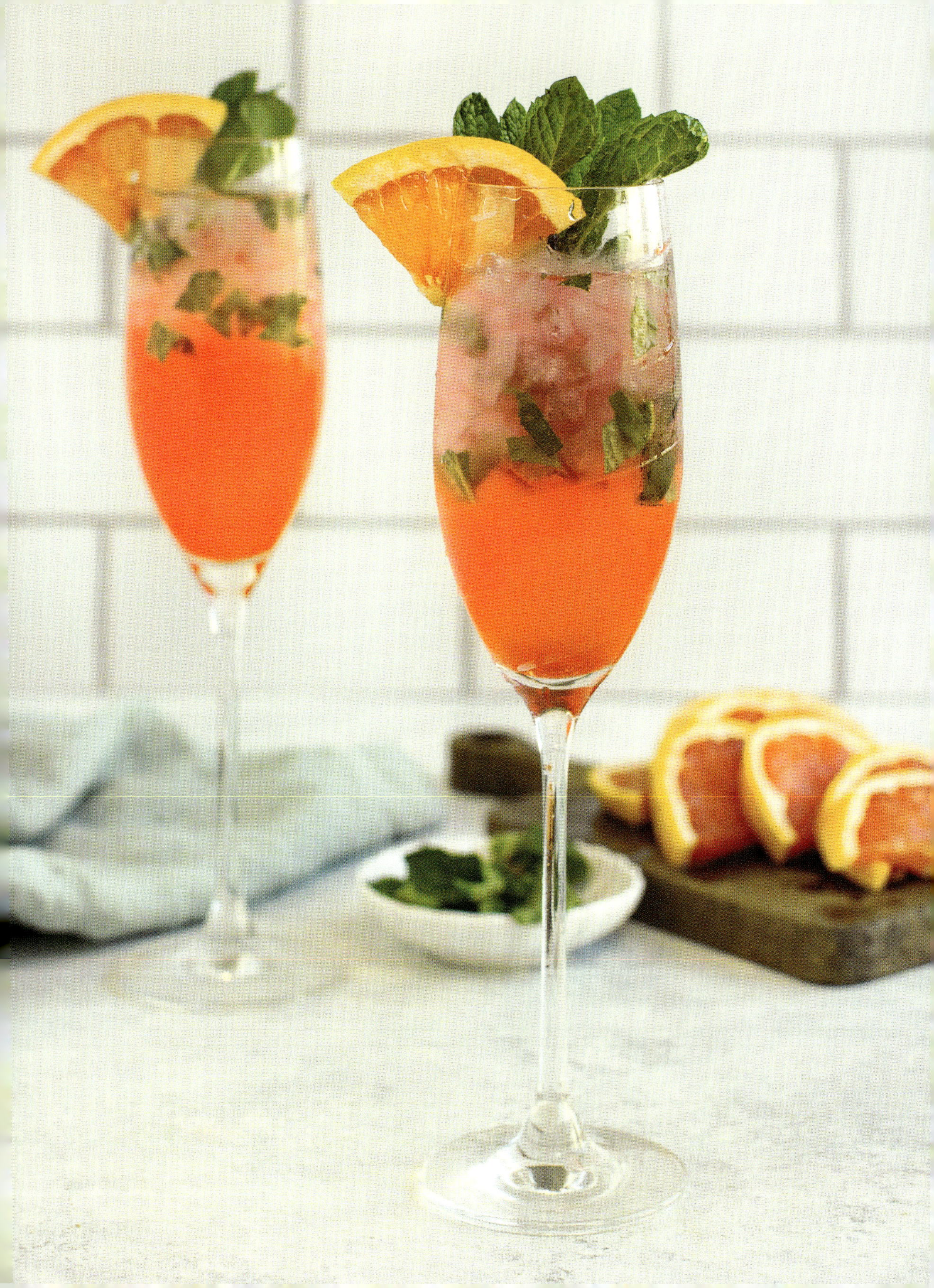

Sparkling Grapefruit Spritzers

An irresistibly rosy hue and hint of fresh mint make these mocktails a satisfying alternative to champagne. If you only have white grapefruit juice, add a drop of grenadine syrup for a pink color.

1 teaspoon chopped fresh mint

1 cup ruby red grapefruit juice

1 (12-ounce) can unflavored seltzer water

1. Divide mint evenly between four champagne flutes.
2. Add ¼ cup (2 ounces) grapefruit juice to each glass, then top with 3 ounces seltzer. Serve immediately.

Serves 4

Per Serving

Calories	25
Fat	0g
Protein	0g
Sodium	14mg
Fiber	0g
Carbohydrates	7g
Sugar	6g

Virgin Mimosas

You'll love these fabulously fizzy Virgin Mimosas. Sparkling white grape juice is sold at most supermarkets and online. If you prefer a traditional mimosa, substitute a bottle of sparkling wine for the white grape juice. For an added kick to the classic cocktail, add a tablespoon of triple sec to each glass.

Serves 8

Per Serving

Calories	78
Fat	0g
Protein	1g
Sodium	6mg
Fiber	0g
Carbohydrates	19g
Sugar	17g

24 ounces freshly squeezed orange juice

1 (750-ml) bottle sparkling white grape juice

1. Pour 3 ounces orange juice into eight champagne flutes.
2. Top with 3 ounces sparkling grape juice in each. Serve immediately.

Make Your Own Sparkling Grape Juice!

If you can't find sparkling grape juice locally, make your own at home. All you'll need is 1 (12-ounce) can of frozen white grape juice concentrate and about 12 ounces of plain seltzer water. Refrigerate the juice concentrate and seltzer, removing once the juice is thawed and the seltzer chilled. Reconstitute the juice according to your specific product's package directions using the seltzer instead of plain water. Stir gently to maximize bubbles.

Ginger Lemonade

There's nothing so refreshing on a hot day as a glass of ice-cold lemonade. In this recipe, the spicy flavor and aroma of fresh ginger adds depth, sophistication, and kick to the beloved classic. Serve immediately or steep in the refrigerator; the longer the lemonade sits, the stronger the ginger becomes.

¼ cup minced fresh ginger

Grated zest of 1 medium lemon

½ cup freshly squeezed lemon juice

4 cups water

½ cup agave nectar

1. Place ginger and lemon zest in a pitcher. Add lemon juice, water, and agave and stir well to combine.
2. Place pitcher in refrigerator and allow lemonade to steep, or serve immediately.
3. When ready to serve, pour lemonade through a fine-mesh sieve into ice-filled glasses. Serve immediately.

Serves 6

Per Serving

Calories	64
Fat	0g
Protein	0g
Sodium	1mg
Fiber	0g
Carbohydrates	16g
Sugar	13g

Ginger Facts

Ginger is the root of a flowering perennial plant. It can be eaten raw, cooked, or ground, and it adds a spicy, distinctive flavor to both sweet and savory dishes. Ginger contains antioxidants believed to improve cognitive ability, inhibit cancer, and prevent cardiovascular disease.

Cranberry Limeade

The cranberry juice and lime used in this Cranberry Limeade are a match made in heaven. Sweet, tart, and tangy, this drink is best served ice-cold.

Serves 4

Per Serving

Calories	91
Fat	0g
Protein	0g
Sodium	2mg
Fiber	0g
Carbohydrates	24g
Sugar	18g

Grated zest of 1 medium lime

1 cup freshly squeezed lime juice

3 cups water

1 cup cranberry juice (100% juice blend)

¼ cup agave nectar

1. Add all ingredients into a small pitcher and stir well to combine.
2. Serve immediately over ice or refrigerate and serve within 2 days.

Mulled Wine

Perfect for winter parties and holiday gatherings, this deliciously steamy, spiked, and spiced combination of red wine and apple cider will keep you and your guests warm and happy. Choose an inexpensive, fruity red wine for this recipe, such as Zinfandel or Merlot.

1 (750-ml) bottle red wine

3 cups apple cider

1 cup apple juice

½ cup triple sec

1 medium navel orange, sliced

1 large red apple, cored and diced

¼ cup fresh whole cranberries, washed and drained

4 whole cinnamon sticks

2 star anise pods

8 whole cloves

1. In a large stockpot, add wine, apple cider, apple juice, and triple sec and stir to combine.
2. Add orange, diced apple, cranberries, cinnamon, star anise, and cloves to pot and stir gently to combine.
3. Place pot over medium-low heat and simmer, stirring frequently, until mixture begins to lightly steam, 15 minutes. You want to warm the wine, not boil the alcohol off!
4. Remove from heat. Ladle into mugs and garnish with some of the fruit. Serve immediately.

Serves 8

Per Serving

Calories	177
Fat	0g
Protein	0g
Sodium	27mg
Fiber	1g
Carbohydrates	20g
Sugar	17g

What Is Star Anise?

Star anise are small, brown, star-shaped seed pods that come from a tree native to China. The pods have an anise or black licorice flavor and are used in many types of cooking. The ground pods are one of the components of the classic Chinese five-spice powder. Try adding a star anise pod to your favorite pot of tea or simmer in a stovetop potpourri.

Maple Mocha Frappé

A creamy concoction of coffee, cocoa, almond milk, and ripe banana, this makes a great breakfast drink or anytime pick-me-up. The stronger the brewed coffee, the more flavor it lends to the frappé. For a fabulous frozen frappé, peel and freeze the bananas ahead of time.

Serves 1

Per Serving

Calories	349
Fat	3g
Protein	5g
Sodium	145mg
Fiber	9g
Carbohydrates	85g
Sugar	53g

2 medium ripe bananas, peeled

3/4 cup brewed coffee, cooled to room temperature

3/4 cup unsweetened almond milk

2 tablespoons pure maple syrup

1 tablespoon plus 1/8 teaspoon unsweetened cocoa powder

1. Place bananas in a food processor and purée.
2. Add coffee, milk, syrup, and 1 tablespoon cocoa powder and pulse until smooth and creamy. Pour into a tall glass and sprinkle with remaining 1/8 teaspoon cocoa powder. Serve immediately.

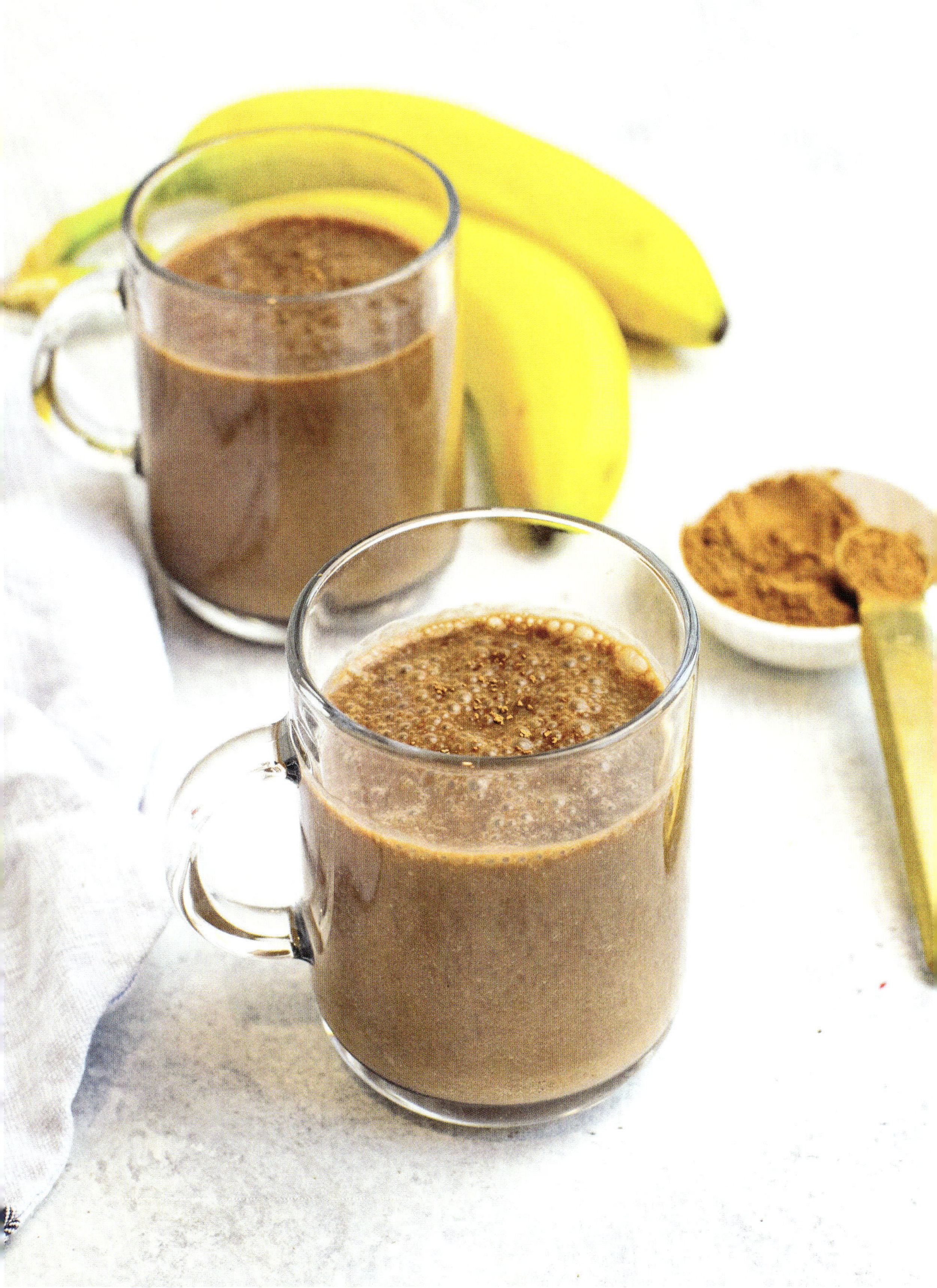

Thin Mint Cocoa

This minty drink is heaven in cocoa form. A healthy vegan version of the traditional treat, this recipe will make your tastebuds tingle.

Serves 4

Per Serving

Calories	145
Fat	2g
Protein	2g
Sodium	137mg
Fiber	3g
Carbohydrates	30g
Sugar	27g

Peppermint Facts

Peppermint is a perennial herb, and its ability to spread and take over a garden is legendary. Its distinctive flavor and tingly freshness enhances drinks, sweets, and salads, as well as many commercial products such as toothpaste. Peppermint is said to soothe upset stomachs, aid with digestion, and protect against cancer.

3½ cups vanilla almond milk
¼ cup unsweetened cocoa powder
¼ cup (unpacked) dark brown sugar
¼ teaspoon peppermint extract

1. In a medium saucepan, add milk and place over medium-high heat.
2. Cook until milk begins to steam, roughly 3–5 minutes, then add cocoa and sugar and whisk well to combine.
3. Remove from heat. Stir in peppermint extract and serve immediately.

Sweet Chai Tea

Basic black tea, oolong tea, or an herbal tea blend such as orange or ginger all work wonderfully in this recipe, so feel free to mix things up! Serve over ice for a refreshing treat in hot weather.

Serves 6

Per Serving

Calories	66
Fat	1g
Protein	0g
Sodium	36mg
Fiber	0g
Carbohydrates	15g
Sugar	13g

5 cups water
1 cup unsweetened almond milk
½ cup agave nectar
1 teaspoon vanilla extract
¼ teaspoon ground cloves
¼ teaspoon ground ginger
⅛ teaspoon ground allspice
⅛ teaspoon ground cardamom
⅛ teaspoon ground cinnamon
6 black tea bags, strings removed

1. In a large saucepan, add water, milk, agave, vanilla, cloves, ginger, allspice, cardamom, and cinnamon and whisk until combined. Add tea bags and stir well.
2. Heat over high heat until contents begin to steam but have not yet boiled, about 5 minutes. Turn off heat and let rest 1 minute.
3. Remove tea bags and ladle into a teapot or mugs. Serve immediately.

Meal Plans

WEEK 1

	Breakfast	Lunch
Day 1	▪ Apple, Banana, and Carrot Muffins Chapter 2 ▪ Nonfat Plain Greek Yogurt	▪ Shrimp with Cocktail Sauce Chapter 3 ▪ Warm Potato Salad with Spinach Chapter 4
Day 2	▪ Apple, Banana, and Carrot Muffins Chapter 2 ▪ Nonfat Plain Greek Yogurt	▪ Chicken Soup with Jalapeño and Lime Chapter 4 ▪ Sweet Corn Muffins Chapter 9
Day 3	▪ Hearty Whole-Grain Breakfast Bowl Chapter 2 ▪ Blueberries ▪ Pistachios	▪ Chicken Soup with Jalapeño and Lime Chapter 4 ▪ Sweet Corn Muffins Chapter 9
Day 4	▪ Lemon Poppy Seed Pancakes Chapter 2 ▪ Vitamin C Juice Chapter 10	▪ Easy Mushroom and Spinach Quiche Chapter 7 ▪ Small Salad—mixed baby greens w/tomatoes and walnuts ▪ Balsamic Vinaigrette Chapter 5
Day 5	▪ Lemon Poppy Seed Pancakes Chapter 2 ▪ Vitamin C Juice Chapter 10 ▪ PB&J Smoothie Chapter 10	▪ Easy Mushroom and Spinach Quiche Chapter 7 ▪ Small Salad—mixed baby greens w/tomatoes and walnuts ▪ Balsamic Vinaigrette Chapter 5
Day 6	▪ Hard-Boiled Egg ▪ Maple Turkey Sausage Chapter 2 ▪ PB&J Smoothie Chapter 10	▪ Roasted Sweet Potato Salad with Kidney Beans and Peas Chapter 4 ▪ Whole Grain Crackers
Day 7	▪ Hard-Boiled Egg ▪ Maple Turkey Sausage Chapter 2	▪ Roasted Sweet Potato Salad with Kidney Beans and Peas Chapter 4 ▪ Whole-Grain Crackers

WEEK 1

	Dinner	Snack/Dessert
Day 1	■ Spaghetti Bolognese Chapter 6	■ Sweet Clementine Salsa Chapter 3 ■ Whole-Grain Tortilla Chips
Day 2	■ Spaghetti Bolognese Chapter 6	■ Sweet Clementine Salsa Chapter 3 ■ Whole-Grain Tortilla Chips
Day 3	■ Salmon with Mango and Chickpea Salad Chapter 6 ■ Whole-Wheat Dinner Roll	■ Foolproof Brownies Chapter 9
Day 4	■ Salmon with Mango and Chickpea Salad Chapter 6 ■ Whole-Wheat Dinner Roll	■ Foolproof Brownies Chapter 9
Day 5	■ Meatless Meatloaf Chapter 7 ■ Perfect Steamed Broccoli Chapter 8	■ Roasted Chickpeas Chapter 3
Day 6	■ Grilled Jerk Chicken Chapter 6 ■ Grilled Pineapple Chapter 9 ■ Brown Rice (1 cup)	■ Roasted Chickpeas Chapter 3
Day 7	■ Grilled Jerk Chicken Chapter 6 ■ Grilled Pineapple Chapter 9 ■ Brown Rice (1 cup)	■ Homemade Banana Ice Cream Chapter 9 ■ Cashews

WEEK 2

	Breakfast	Lunch
Day 1	Whole-Grain Strawberry Muffins Chapter 2 Vitamin A Juice Chapter 10	Tuna Salad with White Beans and Tomatoes Chapter 4
Day 2	Whole-Grain Strawberry Muffins Chapter 2 Vitamin A Juice Chapter 10	Tuna Salad with White Beans and Tomatoes Chapter 4
Day 3	Instant Banana Oatmeal Chapter 2 Walnuts	Oven-Baked Spinach Burgers on whole-wheat buns Chapter 7 Oven-Baked Sweet Potato Fries Chapter 8 Homemade Ketchup Chapter 3
Day 4	Zucchini Muffins Chapter 2 Low-Fat, Low-Sodium Cottage Cheese	Oven-Baked Spinach Burgers on whole-wheat buns Chapter 7 Oven-Baked Sweet Potato Fries Chapter 8 Homemade Ketchup Chapter 5
Day 5	Zucchini Muffins Chapter 2 Low-Fat, Low-Sodium Cottage Cheese	Vegetable Potpie Stew Chapter 4
Day 6	Gingerbread Pancakes Chapter 2	Vegetable Potpie Stew Chapter 4
Day 7	Gingerbread Pancakes Chapter 2	Low-Sodium Caesar Salad Chapter 4 Grilled Salmon

WEEK 2

	Dinner	Snack/Dessert
Day 1	One-Pot Chicken and Vegetables Chapter 6	Chewy Pumpkin Oatmeal Raisin Cookies Chapter 9 Almonds
Day 2	Turkey and Quinoa-Stuffed Peppers Chapter 6	Chewy Pumpkin Oatmeal Raisin Cookies Chapter 9 Almonds
Day 3	Turkey and Quinoa-Stuffed Peppers Chapter 6	Green Pea “Guacamole” Chapter 3 Whole Grain Tortilla Chips
Day 4	Roasted Steelhead Trout with Grapefruit Sauce Chapter 6 Roasted Lemon Asparagus Chapter 8 Quinoa	Green Pea “Guacamole” Chapter 3 Whole-Grain Tortilla Chips
Day 5	Roasted Steelhead Trout with Grapefruit Sauce Chapter 6 Roasted Lemon Asparagus Chapter 8 Quinoa	Cherry Blueberry Crisp Chapter 9 Walnuts
Day 6	Slow Cooker Thai Red Curry Chapter 7 Brown Rice	Crisp and Crunchy Kale Popcorn Chapter 3 Pistachios Bluebaerries
Day 7	Slow Cooker Thai Red Curry Chapter 7 Brown Rice	Crisp and Crunchy Kale Popcorn Chapter 3 Pistachios Blueberries

WEEK 3

	Breakfast	Lunch
Day 1	■ Oven-Baked Apple Pancake **Chapter 9**	■ Vegetable Pasta Salad with Zesty Italian Dressing **Chapter 4**
Day 2	■ Scrambled Egg ■ Maple Turkey Sausage **Chapter 2** ■ Maple Mocha Frappé **Chapter 10**	■ Vegetable Pasta Salad with Zesty Italian Dressing **Chapter 4**
Day 3	■ Scrambled Egg ■ Maple Turkey Sausage **Chapter 2** ■ Maple Mocha Frappé **Chapter 10**	■ Slow Cooker Split Pea Soup **Chapter 4** ■ Whole Grain Roll
Day 4	■ Instant Peaches and Cream Oatmeal **Chapter 2** ■ Almonds	■ Slow Cooker Split Pea Soup **Chapter 4** ■ Whole-Grain Roll
Day 5	■ Peanut Butter and Jelly Pancakes **Chapter 2**	■ Mandarin Chicken Salad with Spinach and Pecans **Chapter 4** ■ Whole-Grain Roll
Day 6	■ Peanut Butter and Jelly Pancakes **Chapter 2**	■ Tasty Lentil Tacos **Chapter 7**
Day 7	■ Hearty Whole-Grain Breakfast Bowl **Chapter 2** ■ Blueberries ■ Walnuts	■ Tasty Lentil Tacos **Chapter 7**

WEEK 3

	Dinner	Snack/Dessert
Day 1	■ Spicy Pan-Roasted Chickpeas with Tahini Sauce **Chapter 7**	■ Cilantro Lime Black Bean Spread **Chapter 3** ■ Whole-Grain Pita Chips ■ Blueberries
Day 2	■ Spicy Pan-Roasted Chickpeas with Tahini Sauce **Chapter 7**	■ Cilantro Lime Black Bean Spread **Chapter 3** ■ Whole-Grain Pita Chips ■ Blueberries
Day 3	■ Quick Vegan Pizza **Chapter 7** ■ Small Salad—mixed baby greens w/tomatoes ■ Tomato Garlic Dressing **Chapter 5**	■ Jam-Filled Cupcakes **Chapter 9** ■ Air-Popped Popcorn
Day 4	■ Baked Tuna Cakes **Chapter 6** ■ Baked Spinach and Pea Risotto **Chapter 8** ■ Oven-Roasted Cherry Tomatoes **Chapter 8**	■ Jam-Filled Cupcakes **Chapter 9** ■ Air-Popped Popcorn
Day 5	■ Baked Tuna Cakes **Chapter 6** ■ Baked Spinach and Pea Risotto **Chapter 8** ■ Oven-Roasted Cherry Tomatoes **Chapter 8**	■ Mango Salsa **Chapter 5** ■ Whole-Grain Tortilla Chips
Day 6	■ Slow Cooker Chicken with Butternut Squash and Kale **Chapter 6** ■ Quinoa	■ Mango Salsa **Chapter 5** ■ Whole-Grain Tortilla Chips
Day 7	■ Slow Cooker Chicken with Butternut Squash and Kale **Chapter 6** ■ Quinoa	■ Chocolate-Drizzled Almond Biscotti **Chapter 9**

WEEK 4

	Breakfast	Lunch
Day 1	Vegetable Hash Chapter 2 Homemade Vegtable Juice Chapter 10	Low-Sodium Greek Salad Chapter 4 Grilled Chicken Breast Whole-Grain Roll
Day 2	Vegetable Hash Chapter 2 Homemade Vegetable Juice Chapter 10	Homemade Black Bean Burgers Chapter 7 Sweet and Tangy Coleslaw with Jalapeño and Lime Chapter 4
Day 3	Hearty Whole-Grain Breakfast Bowl Chapter 2 Blueberries Walnuts	Homemade Black Bean Burgers Chapter 7 Sweet and Tangy Coleslaw with Jalapeño and Lime Chapter 4
Day 4	Blueberry Lemon Corn Bread Chapter 2 Nonfat Greek Yogurt	Salmon Salad with Whole-Wheat Couscous and Dill Chapter 4
Day 5	Blueberry Lemon Corn Bread Chapter 2 Nonfat Greek Yogurt	Slow Cooker Sweet Potato and Kale Stew Chapter 4
Day 6	Hard-Boiled Egg Peppery Apple Chicken Sausage Chapter 2 Creamy "Milk" Shake Chapter 10	Slow Cooker Sweet Potato and Kale Stew Chapter 4
Day 7	Hard-Boiled Egg Peppery Apple Chicken Sausage Chapter 2 Creamy "Milk" Shake Chapter 10	Roasted Beets with Chili Lime Vinaigrette Chapter 8 Grilled Shrimp Whole-Grain Roll

WEEK 4

	Dinner	Snack/Dessert
Day 1	■ Scallops Fra Diavolo Chapter 6 ■ Whole-Wheat Linguine (1 cup) ■ Sweet and Spicy Brussels Sprouts Chapter 8	■ Chocolate-Drizzled Almond Biscotti Chapter 9
Day 2	■ Scallops Fra Diavolo Chapter 6 ■ Whole-Wheat Linguine (1 cup) ■ Sweet and Spicy Brussels Sprouts Chapter 8	■ Basil Pesto Hummus Chapter 3 ■ Whole-Grain Pita Chips
Day 3	■ Spicy Chickpea Tacos with Arugula Chapter 7	■ Basil Pesto Hummus Chapter 3 ■ Whole-Grain Pita Chips
Day 4	■ Spicy Chickpea Tacos with Arugula Chapter 7	■ Party Mix Popcorn Chapter 3 ■ Avocado Whip with Carrots Chapter 5
Day 5	■ Chicken Cacciatore Chapter 6 ■ Whole-Wheat Pasta (1 cup) ■ Small Salad—mixed baby greens w/tomatoes ■ Balsamic Vinaigrette Chapter 5	■ Party Mix Popcorn Chapter 3 ■ Avocado Whip with Carrots Chapter 5
Day 6	■ Chicken Cacciatore Chapter 6 ■ Whole-Wheat Pasta (1 cup) ■ Small Salad—mixed baby greens w/tomatoes ■ Balsamic Vinaigrette Chapter 5	■ Chocolate Gingerbread Chapter 9 ■ Walnuts
Day 7	■ Savory Stuffed Acorn Squash Chapter 7 ■ Quinoa	■ Chocolate Gingerbread Chapter 9 ■ Walnuts

STANDARD US/METRIC MEASUREMENT CONVERSIONS

VOLUME CONVERSIONS

US Volume Measure	Metric Equivalent
⅛ teaspoon	0.5 milliliter
¼ teaspoon	1 milliliter
½ teaspoon	2 milliliters
1 teaspoon	5 milliliters
½ tablespoon	7 milliliters
1 tablespoon (3 teaspoons)	15 milliliters
2 tablespoons (1 fluid ounce)	30 milliliters
¼ cup (4 tablespoons)	60 milliliters
⅓ cup	90 milliliters
½ cup (4 fluid ounces)	125 milliliters
⅔ cup	160 milliliters
¾ cup (6 fluid ounces)	180 milliliters
1 cup (16 tablespoons)	250 milliliters
1 pint (2 cups)	500 milliliters
1 quart (4 cups)	1 liter (about)

WEIGHT CONVERSIONS

US Weight Measure	Metric Equivalent
½ ounce	15 grams
1 ounce	30 grams
2 ounces	60 grams
3 ounces	85 grams
¼ pound (4 ounces)	115 grams
½ pound (8 ounces)	225 grams
¾ pound (12 ounces)	340 grams
1 pound (16 ounces)	454 grams

OVEN TEMPERATURE CONVERSIONS

Degrees Fahrenheit	Degrees Celsius
200 degrees F	95 degrees C
250 degrees F	120 degrees C
275 degrees F	135 degrees C
300 degrees F	150 degrees C
325 degrees F	160 degrees C
350 degrees F	180 degrees C
375 degrees F	190 degrees C
400 degrees F	205 degrees C
425 degrees F	220 degrees C
450 degrees F	230 degrees C

BAKING PAN SIZES

American	Metric
8 × 1½ inch round baking pan	20 × 4 cm cake tin
9 × 1½ inch round baking pan	23 × 3.5 cm cake tin
11 × 7 × 1½ inch baking pan	28 × 18 × 4 cm baking tin
13 × 9 × 2 inch baking pan	30 × 20 × 5 cm baking tin
2 quart rectangular baking dish	30 × 20 × 3 cm baking tin
15 × 10 × 2 inch baking pan	30 × 25 × 2 cm baking tin (Swiss roll tin)
9 inch pie plate	22 × 4 or 23 × 4 cm pie plate
7 or 8 inch springform pan	18 or 20 cm springform or loose bottom cake tin
9 × 5 × 3 inch loaf pan	23 × 13 × 7 cm or 2 lb narrow loaf or pate tin
1½ quart casserole	1.5 liter casserole
2 quart casserole	2 liter casserole

Index